Analyzing Rater Agreement

Manifest Variable Methods

Analyzing Rater Agreement

Manifest Variable Methods

Alexander von Eye
Michigan State University

Eun Young Mun
University of Alabama at Birmingham

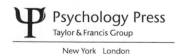
Psychology Press
Taylor & Francis Group

New York   London

Camera ready copy for this book was provided by the authors.

First published by
Lawrence Erlbaum Associates, Inc., Publishers
10 Industrial Avenue
Mahwah, New Jersey 07430

This edition published 2012 by Psychology Press

Psychology Press
Taylor & Francis Group
711 Third Avenue
New York, NY 10017

Psychology Press
Taylor & Francis Group
27 Church Road, Hove
East Sussex BN3 2FA

Cover design by Kathryn Houghtaling Lacey

Library of Congress Cataloging-in-Publication Data

Eye, Alexander von.
    Analyzing rater agreement: manifest variable methods / Alexander von Eye, Eun Young Mun.
        p. cm.

Includes bibliographical references and index.

ISBN 0-8058-4967-X (alk. paper)
   1. Multivariate analysis. 2. Acquiescence (Psychology)—Statistical methods. I. Mun, Eun Young. II. Title.
QA278.E94 2004
519.5'35—dc22
                                    2004043344
                                          CIP

Contents

4.   Correlation Structures   115

5.   Computer Applications   131

Supplementary Resources Disclaimer

Additional resources were previously made available for this title on CD. However, as CD has become a less accessible format, all resources have been moved to a more convenient online download option.

You can find these resources available here: www.routledge.com/9780805849677

Please note: Where this title mentions the associated disc, please use the downloadable resources instead.

Preface

Agreement among raters is of great importance in many domains, both academic and nonacademic. In the Olympic Games, the medals and ranking in gymnastics, figure skating, synchronized swimming, and other disciplines are based on the ratings of several judges. Extreme judgements are often discarded from the pool of scores used for the ranking. In medicine, diagnoses are often provided by more than one doctor, to make sure the proposed treatment is optimal. In criminal trials, a group of jurors is used, and sentencing depends, among other things, on the complete agreement among the jurors. In observational studies, researchers increase reliability by discussing discrepant ratings. Restaurants receive Michelin stars only after several test-eaters agree on the chef's performance. There are many more examples.

We believe that this book will appeal to a broad range of students and researchers, in particular in the areas of psychology, biostatistics, medical research, education anthropology, sociology, and many other areas in which ratings are provided by multiple sources. A large number of models is presented, and examples are provided from many of these fields and disciplines.

This text describes four approaches to the statistical analysis of rater agreement. The first approach, covered in chapter 1, involves calculating coefficients that allow one to summarize agreement in a single score. Five coefficients are reviewed that differ in (1) the scale level of rating categories that they can analyze; (2) the assumptions made when specifying a chance model, that is, the model with which the observed agreement is compared; (3) whether or not there exist significance tests; and (4) whether they allow one to place weights on rating categories.

The second approach, presented in chapter 2, involves estimating log-linear models. These are typically more complex than coefficients of rater agreement, and allow one to test specific hypotheses about the structure of a cross-classification of two or more raters' judgements. Often, such cross-classifications display characteristics such as, for instance, trends, that help interpret the joint frequency distribution of two or more raters. This text presents a family of log-linear models and discusses submodels, that is, special cases.

The third approach, in chapter 3, involves exploring cross-classifications or raters' agreement for indicators of agreement or disagreement, and for indicators of such characteristics as trends. Methods of Configural Frequency Analysis are discussed for the exploration of cross-classification. These methods allow one to identify where exactly in a table there is beyond chance agreement and where there is beyond chance lack of agreement.

The approach in chapter 4 examines rater agreement taking a different perspective from the first three approaches. Specifically, this approach compares the correlation or covariation structures of variables that raters use to describe objects, behaviors, or individuals. These structures can be compared for two or more raters.

Chapter 5 covers computer applications. Most of the models discussed in the contexts of coefficients of rater agreement, log-linear modeling, and structural modeling can be tested using commercial software such as SPSS®, SYSTAT®, and LISREL®. For some of the approaches to analyzing rater agreement, more specialized programs are needed. This applies in particular to the Configural Frequency Analysis program that is needed for exploration of agreement tables. This program is available free of charge.

All of the methods presented in this text operate at the manifest variable level, that is, at the level of observed variables. A number of latent variable and factor models exist for the analysis of rater agreement. These models assume that unmeasured, latent variables exist that determine raters' judgements. However, with the goals of (1) keeping this text compact and (2) reflecting the vast majority of applications, the methods discussed here in detail and the examples all operate at the manifest variable level.

This book also contains a series of exercises for each chapter. Thus, the book may be useful for use in class. An additional set of exercises is provided on the companion CD. The CD not only presents the exercises and the solutions, but also shows, step-by-step, how to solve the exercises using the software that is presented in chapter 5.

Readers will benefit most from this text if their exposure to statistics includes χ^2-methods and the matrix approach to regression analysis. Additional knowledge of log-linear modeling will make this text easy reading.

Acknowledgments

We are indebted to a number of people, each of whom supported us in his or her own way. First, there are the reviewers of a first draft who encouraged us and suggested a number of changes and additions. Each of these clearly improved the text. Second, there are Debra Riegert and Lawrence Erlbaum of LEA who supported this project from the very moment we approached them, and LEA's Barbara Wieghaus who did a marvelous editing job. Third, there are our families. We agree in the high ratings we give to Donata, Maxi, Valerie, and Julian, and to Feng. Without you, life would not be half as nice and interesting.

Alexander von Eye & Eun Young Mun

1.   Coefficients of Rater Agreement

The number of coefficients for rater agreement is large. However, the number of coefficients that is actually used in empirical research is small. The present section discusses five of the more frequently used coefficients. The first is Cohen's (1960) κ (kappa), one of the most widely employed coefficients in the social sciences. κ is a coefficient for nominal level variables. The second and the third coefficients are variants of κ. The second coefficient, weighted κ, allows the statistical analyst to place differential weights on discrepant ratings. This coefficient requires ordinal rating scales. The third coefficient is Brennan and Prediger's $κ_n$, a variant of κ that uses a different chance model than the original κ. The fourth coefficient is raw agreement which expresses the degree of agreement as percentage of judgements in which raters agree. The fifth coefficient discussed here is Kendall's W. This coefficient is defined for ordinal variables.

1.1   Cohen's κ (Kappa)

Clearly the most frequently used coefficient of rater agreement is Cohen's (1960) kappa, κ. In its original form, which is presented in this section, this coefficient can be applied to square cross-classifications of two raters' judgements (variants for three or more raters are presented in Section 1.6). These cross-classifications are also called *agreement tables*. Consider the two raters A and B who used the three categories 1, 2, and 3 to evaluate students' performance in English. The cross-classification of these raters' judgements can be depicted as given in Table 1.1.

The interpretation of the frequencies, m_{ij}, in the cross-classification given in Table 1.1 is straightforward. Cell 11 displays the number of instances in which both Rater A and Rater B used Category 1. Cell 12 contains the number of instances in which Rater A used Category 1 and Rater B used Category 2, and so forth. The cells with indexes $i = j$ display the numbers of incidences in which the two raters used the same category. These cells are also called the *agreement cells*. These cells are shaded in Table 1.1.

Table 1.1:   Cross-Classification of Two Raters' Judgements

		Rater B Rating Categories		
		1	2	3
Rater A Rating Categories	1	m_{11}	m_{12}	m_{13}
	2	m_{21}	m_{22}	m_{23}
	3	m_{31}	m_{32}	m_{33}

The following two sections first introduce κ as a coefficient that allows one to describe rater agreement in the form of a summary statement for an entire table. Second, *conditional* κ is introduced. This measure allows one to describe rater agreement separately for each rating category.

1.1.1 κ as a Summary Statement for the Entire Agreement Table

To introduce Cohen's κ, let p_{ij} be the probability of Cell ij. The cells that indicate rater agreement, that is, the *agreement cells*, have probability p_{ii}. The parameter theta$_1$,

$$\theta_1 = \sum_{i=1}^{I} p_{ii}$$

describes the proportion of instances in which the two raters agree, where I is the number of categories. To have a reference with which θ_1 can be compared, we assume independence of the two raters. In other words, we assume that the raters did not influence each other when evaluating the students. (Later in this text, we will see that this assumption corresponds to main effects models in log-linear analysis and Configural Frequency Analysis.) Based on this assumption, we can estimate the proportion of instances in which the two raters agree by chance using theta$_2$,

$$\theta_2 = \sum_{i=1}^{I} p_{i.}\, p_{.i} \, ,$$

where a period indicate the marginal summed across. More specifically, $i.$ indicates the ith row total and $.i$ indicates the ith column total. Subtracting θ_2 from θ_1 results in a measure of rater agreement, corrected by chance. If the difference $\theta_1 - \theta_2$ is positive, the two raters agree more often than expected based on chance. If $\theta_1 - \theta_2$ is negative, they agree less often than expected based on chance.

The largest possible discrepancy between θ_1 and θ_2 is $1 - \theta_2$. This discrepancy results when all judgements appear in the shaded cells of the cross-classification, that is, the agreement cells of the cross-classification (see Table 1.1). In this case, agreement is perfect. Weighting the difference $\theta_1 - \theta_2$ by $1 - \theta_2$ yields Cohen's κ (kappa),

$$\kappa = \frac{\theta_1 - \theta_2}{1 - \theta_2} \, .$$

κ indicates the proportion of incidences in which two raters use the same categories to evaluate a number of objects, corrected by chance.

A general interpretation of κ focuses on the characteristic of κ as a measure of *proportionate reduction in error* (PRE; Fleiss, 1975). κ inspects the cells in the main diagonal of the I x I cross-classification of two raters' judgements. The question asked is how the observed frequency distribution differs from the expected, or chance distribution in the diagonal cells. If the observed distribution contains more cases of agreement, one expresses the result in terms of the proportionate reduction in error. This reduction indicates that the observed frequency distribution contains more cases of agreement and fewer cases of disagreement than the chance distribution. In different terms, κ is an example of a PRE measure of the form

$$PRE = \frac{\theta_1 - \theta_2}{\max(\theta_1) - \theta_2} \, .$$

The maximum value that θ_1 can take is 1. This would indicate that all responses are located in the main diagonal or, that there are no disagreements. The above definition of κ uses $\theta_1 = 1$ in the denominator. Thus, κ can be identified as a PRE measure.

An estimate of κ under a multinomial sampling scheme can be obtained by kappa hat,

$$\hat{\kappa} = \frac{N \sum_i m_{ii} - \sum_i m_{i.} m_{.i}}{N^2 - \sum_i m_{i.} m_{.i}},$$

where $i = 1, ..., I$ indexes the categories used by the raters, N is the number of decisions made by the raters, and m indicates the observed frequencies. This measure has been used and discussed extensively (for an overview see, e.g., Agresti, 2002; Wickens, 1989). Historically, κ can be traced back to λ, a measure of asymmetric similarity (Goodman, & Kruskal, 1954; cf. Froman & Llabre, 1985).

The characteristics of κ include

(1)   The range of κ is $-\infty < \kappa \leq 1$; the smallest possible value of κ is, for a sample of size N, $1 - \dfrac{N}{1 - \sum_i m_{ii}}$, where m_{ii} is the frequency in Cell ii, that is, an agreement cell (in the main diagonal). Positive values of κ indicate agreement better than chance, and negative values of κ indicate agreement less than chance.

(2) $\kappa = 0$ if the probability of disagreement (off-diagonal cells) is the same as the probability of agreement (diagonal cells); κ can be zero even if the raters' judgements are not independent.

(3) $\kappa = 1$ only if the probability in the disagreement cells is zero.

(4) κ is defined only if at least two categories are used by both raters, that is, if the probability, p_{ij}, is greater than zero for at least two cells.

(5)   If the probability in the off-diagonals is non-zero, the maximum value of κ decreases as the marginals deviate from a uniform distribution (see the notion of *prevalence dependency* of chance-corrected agreement; Guggenmoos-Holzmann, 1995).

(6)   When the probability of disagreement decreases and is smaller than the number of agreements, κ increases monotonically (see Figure 1, below); when the probability of disagreement increases and is

greater than the probability of agreement, κ does not decrease monotonically (see Figure 2, below; von Eye & Sörensen, 1991). Multiplied by 100, κ indicates the percentage by which two raters' agreement exceeds the agreement that could be expected from chance.

(7)

A number of significance tests has been proposed for κ. Formulas for estimators of standard errors for κ can be found, for instance in Liebetrau (1983) and in Hildebrand et al. (1977b). When the sample is sufficiently large, $\hat{\kappa}$ is approximately normally distributed with mean κ. The standard error of $\hat{\kappa}$ is σ_κ (sigma$_{\text{kappa}}$),

$$\sigma_{\hat{\kappa}} = \sqrt{\frac{1}{N(1 - \theta_2)^2} \left[\theta_2 + \theta_2^2 - \sum_{i=1}^{I} p_{i.} \, p_{.i} \, (p_{i.} + p_{.i}) \right]}$$

(Fleiss, Cohen, & Everitt, 1969). When estimating the standard error from empirical data, one uses $\hat{p}_{ij} = \dfrac{m_{ij}}{N}$ to estimate p_{ij}, $\hat{p}_{i.}$ to estimate $p_{i.}$, and $\hat{p}_{.i}$ to estimate $p_{.i}$.

A significance test for κ can then use the approximately standard normally distributed

$$z_\kappa = \frac{\hat{\kappa}}{\hat{\sigma}_{\hat{\kappa}}},$$

where the denominator is estimated as given above. As an alternative to the z-test, von Eye and Brandtstädter (1988a) proposed using the binomial test. This test will be discussed in more detail in the contexts of agreement among three or more raters (Section 1.6) and exploratory analysis of rater agreement (Section 3.1).

In addition to discussing significance tests, a number of authors has proposed guidelines for the interpretation of κ. Unfortunately, these guidelines are contradictory. For example, Landis and Koch (1977) propose the interpretation

- $\kappa < 0.00$ poor agreement
- $0.00 \le \kappa \le 0.20$ slight
- $0.21 \le \kappa \le 0.40$ fair
- $0.41 \le \kappa \le 0.60$ moderate
- $0.61 \le \kappa \le 0.80$ substantial, and
- $0.81 \le \kappa \le 1.00$ almost perfect agreement.

In contrast, Fleiss (1981) suggests the categories

- $\kappa < 0.40$ poor agreement
- $0.40 \leq \kappa \leq 0.75$ good, and
- $\kappa > 0.75$ excellent agreement.

Thus, researchers using such guidelines should make explicit which guidelines they refer to. It is well known that even small values of κ can be significant if the sample is large. Therefore, researchers typically report (1) κ itself, (2) the results from significance tests, and (3) other estimates such as the coefficient of raw agreement (see Section 1.3).

Data example. The following data example, taken from von Eye and Schuster (2000) describes results from a study on the reliability of psychiatric diagnoses. Two psychiatrists re-evaluated the files of $N = 129$ inpatients that had previously been diagnosed as clinically depressed. The psychiatrists evaluated the severity of the patients' depression. The rating categories were 1 = not depressed, 2 = mildly depressed, and 3 = clinically depressed. The data in Table 1.2 describe the ratings that the two raters provided. In the following analysis, we ask (1) whether the two raters agree beyond chance, and (2) whether the agreement is statistically significantly greater than could be expected from chance.

Table 1.2: Two Psychiatrists' Perception of Severity of Depression (estimated expected cell frequencies *in italics*)

		Psychiatrist 2: Severity of Depression			Row Sums
		1	2	3	
Psychiatrist 1: Severity of Depression	1	11 *2.98*	2 *3.22*	19 *25.80*	32
	2	1 *0.65*	3 *0.71*	3 *5.64*	7
	3	0 *8.37*	8 *9.07*	82 *72.56*	90
Column Sums		12	13	104	N = 129

Table 1.2 displays both the observed and the expected cell frequencies for each cell. The expected frequencies are printed in italics, right under the observed frequencies. The expected cell frequencies can be calculated using the programs illustrated in Chapter 5. For the unweighted κ, the same methods as for the standard χ^2 can be used. Specifically, the expected frequency for Cell ij can be estimated by

$$\hat{m}_{ij} = \frac{m_{i.} m_{.j}}{N} ,$$

where $m_{i.}$ indicates the row totals and $m_{.j}$ indicates the column totals. For example, the expected frequency for Cell 11 can be estimated as $e_{11} = (32 \cdot 12) / 129 = 2.977$.

For each of the tables under study, the Pearson X^2 or the likelihood ratio X^2 can be estimated to determine whether the variables that span the agreement table are independent. The Pearson X^2 is calculated as

$$X^2 = \sum_{ij} \frac{(m_{ij} - \hat{m}_{ij})^2}{\hat{m}_{ij}}$$

The likelihood ratio X^2, which is often preferred when hierarchically related models are compared, is

$$LR\text{-}X^2 = 2\sum_{ij} m_{ij} \log_e \frac{m_{ij}}{\hat{m}_{ij}}$$

Both the Pearson X^2 and the $LR\text{-}X^2$ are distributed approximately as χ^2 with $df = IJ - (I - 1) - (J - 1) - 1$. This applies accordingly for tables for three or more raters.

We calculate for Table 1.2 a goodness-of-fit Likelihood Ratio X^2 = 39.03 ($df = 4$; $p < 0.01$) and

$$\hat{\kappa} = \frac{129 \cdot 96 - (12 \cdot 32 + 13 \cdot 7 + 104 \cdot 90)}{129^2 - (12 \cdot 32 + 13 \cdot 7 + 104 \cdot 90)} = 0.375$$

($\hat{se}_\kappa = 0.079$; $z = 4.747$; $p < 0.01$). The proportion that the two psychiatrists agreed was 0.744 (that is, $\hat{\theta}_1 = (11+3+82) / 129 = 0.744$). The proportion of chance agreement was 0.591 (that is, $\hat{\theta}_2 = (2.98+0.71+72.56) / 129 = 0.591$). The coefficient κ is a ratio of improvement over chance, relative to the maximally possible improvement, or $\hat{\kappa} = (0.744 - 0.591) / (1 - 0.591) = 0.375$. We thus conclude (1) from the Likelihood Ratio X^2, that the assumption of independence between these two raters' perceptions can be rejected; (2) from κ, that the raters' agreement is 37.5% greater than was expected based on chance; and (3) from z that the agreement between the two raters is significantly better than chance.

1.1.2   Conditional κ

The form in which κ was presented in Section 1.1.1 is that of a summary statement for the entire agreement table. As such, it describes the degree of agreement beyond chance, aggregated over all rating categories. It goes without saying that a particular value of κ does not imply that agreement is equally strong for each rating category. In fact, it is conceivable that agreement is positive for some categories and negative for others, or that raters agree strongly in extreme categories but only weakly or not at all in less extreme categories. Therefore, a κ-like measure that can be estimated separately for each rating category could be of use. Such a measure was proposed by Coleman (1966) and Light (1969).[1]

Specifically, the authors proposed a measure of agreement for those cases in which the rater that is used to define the rows of an agreement table assigns the ith category. Let, as before, p_{ii} be the probability of cell ii in the agreement table, $p_{i.}$ the probability that the first rater (rows) uses Category i, and $p_{.i}$ the probability that the second rater (columns) also uses Category i. Then, a κ measure for rating category i is kappa$_i$,

$$\kappa_i = \frac{\dfrac{p_{ii}}{p_{i.}} - p_{.i}}{1 - p_{.i}} = \frac{p_{ii} - p_{i.}p_{.i}}{p_{i.} - p_{i.}p_{.i}}$$

This measure is known as *conditional* κ or as *partial* κ. The sampling scheme for partial κ is the same as for the aggregate κ. It typically is multinomial. That is, only the sample size, N, is fixed. Were row or column marginals fixed, the sampling scheme would be product multinomial. Under a multinomial sampling scheme, partial κ can be estimated by

$$\hat{\kappa}_i = \frac{Nm_{ii} - m_{i.}m_{.i}}{Nm_{i.} - m_{i.}m_{.i}},$$

where N and the quantities m are defined as before. Under the base model of independence, that is, under the model that is typically employed to

---

[1] The Coleman and Light references are cited from Bishop, Fienberg, and Holland (1975). We did not have access to these sources.

estimate the expected cell frequencies for the aggregate measure κ, the asymptotic variance of the partial κ_i is

$$\sigma_i^2 = \frac{1}{N} \frac{p_{.i}(1 - p_{i.})}{p_{i.}(1 - p_{.i})} .$$

This variance can be estimated from the data by

$$s_i^2 = \frac{1}{N} \frac{\dfrac{m_{.i}}{N}\left(1 - \dfrac{m_{i.}}{N}\right)}{\dfrac{m_{i.}}{N}\left(1 - \dfrac{m_{.i}}{N}\right)} .$$

Using κ_i and this variance estimate, one can test the null hypothesis that κ_i = 0 by means of

$$z_i = \frac{\kappa_i}{s_i} .$$

The variance estimate can also be used to estimated confidence bounds for κ_i.

Data example. The two psychiatrists who rated 129 patient files as to the degree of the patients' depression (data in Table 1.2) agreed 37.5% better than chance. This proportionate increase in hits was significant. We now ask (1) whether this aggregate score describes the two raters' agreement equally well for each category, and (2) whether the two raters' agreement is significant for each category.

The first estimate of the three partial κ-scores is calculated as

$$\hat{\kappa}_1 = \frac{129 \cdot 11 - 129 \cdot 2.98}{129 \cdot 32 - 129 \cdot 2.98} = 0.276.$$

Accordingly, the estimates for the second and the third partial κ-scores are $\hat{\kappa}_2 = 0.365$, and $\hat{\kappa}_3 = 0.541$. Obviously, the partial κ-scores suggest that the two psychiatrists do not agree equally in the three degrees of depression. Their agreement is weakest in Category 1, that is, the category 'not depressed,' and strongest in the Category 3, that is, the category 'clinically depressed.' The estimates of the three variances are $s_1^2 = 0.002$, $s_2^2 = 0.015$, and $s_3^2 = 0.014$. The three z-scores are then $z_1 = 5.62$, $z_2 = 2.97$, and $z_3 = 4.58$. We thus reject all three null hypotheses of no

agreement beyond chance between the two psychiatrists for depression
severity i.

1.2   Weighted κ

It is one of the main characteristics of κ that each discrepancy between two
judgements is weighted equally. For example, the discrepancy between two
ratings of *not depressed* (= 1) and *clinically depressed* (= 3) carries the
same weight as the discrepancy between *mildly depressed* (= 2) and
clinically depressed (= 3). To allow for weights that make it possible to
take into account the magnitude of discrepancy, Cohen (1968) introduced
weighted κ. Proceeding as in Section 1.1, we define theta$_1$* as

$$\theta_1^* = \sum_{i=1}^{I} \sum_{j=1}^{J} \omega_{ij}\, P_{ij}$$

and theta$_2$* as

$$\theta_2^* = \sum_{i=1}^{I} \sum_{j=1}^{J} \omega_{ij}\, P_{i.}\, P_{.j}\, ,$$

where the ω_{ij} (omega$_{ij}$) are the weights. Cohen requires for these weights
that

(1) $0 \le \omega_{ij} \le 1$, and
(2)   they be ratios.

The second requirement means that a weight of $\omega_{ij} = 0.5$ indicates
agreement that weighs twice that of $\omega_{ij} = 0.25$. Using the parameters θ_1^*
and θ_2^*, one can define a weighted κ as

$$\kappa_w = \frac{\theta_1^* - \theta_2^*}{1 - \theta_2^*}\, .$$

The minimum value of κ_w is $-\dfrac{\theta_2^*}{1 - \theta_2^*}$. The maximum value is still 1. In
explicit form, an estimate of weighted κ is

$$\hat{\kappa}_w = \frac{N \sum_i \sum_j \omega_{ij} m_{ij} - \sum_i \sum_j \omega_{ij} m_{i.} m_{.j}}{N^2 - \sum_i \sum_j \omega_{ij} m_{i.} m_{.j}}$$

Under the null hypothesis that $\kappa_w = 0$, its standard error is

$$\sigma_{\kappa_w} = \sqrt{\frac{1}{N(1 - \theta_2^*)^2} \left[\sum_i \sum_j P_{i.} P_{.j} \omega_{ij} - (\overline{\omega}_{i.} + \overline{\omega}_{.j})]^2 - \theta_2^{*2} \right]},$$

with

$$\overline{\omega}_{i.} = \sum_j \omega_{ij} P_{.j},$$

and

$$\overline{\omega}_{.j} = \sum_i \omega_{ij} P_{i.}$$

In a fashion analogous to the original unweighted κ, the null hypothesis that the weighted κ is equal to zero, can be tested using the z-statistic

$$z_{\kappa_w} = \frac{\hat{\kappa}_w}{\hat{\sigma}_{\hat{\kappa}_w}},$$

where the denominator is estimated as indicated above.

It is easy to show that κ is a special case of κ_w. κ can be considered a case where researchers set the weight $\omega_{ij} = 0$ for all forms of disagreement and $\omega_{ii} = 1$ for all cases of agreement, or

$$\omega_{ij} = \begin{cases} 1 & if\ i = j \\ 0 & if\ i \neq j \end{cases}.$$

If the weights are selected according to this scheme, $\kappa = \kappa_w$.

Data example. For the following example, we use the psychiatric data from Table 1.2 again. We now place weights on the data such that

- the two psychiatrists are considered in full agreement if $i = j$; in these cases, we assign $\omega_{ii} = 1$;
- the two psychiatrists are considered in partial agreement if the

discrepancy between their ratings does not go beyond directly adjacent rating categories; that is, we assign $\omega_{ij} = 0.5$, if $|i - j| = 1$; and

the two psychiatrists are considered in disagreement if the discrepancy between their ratings does go beyond directly adjacent rating categories; that is, we assign $\omega_{ij} = 0$, if $|i - j| > 1$.

The weights that result from these specifications appear in Table 1.3. Obviously, defining partial agreement weights in this fashion requires rating categories at the ordinal scale level.

The expected cell frequencies for the calculation of the weighted κ_w are the same as for the unweighted κ, and so is the overall goodness-of-fit Likelihood Ratio X^2. However, the value for κ_w differs from the value for κ. Specifically, we calculate $\kappa_w = 0.402$. The tail probability for this score is $p = 0.0006$. We thus conclude that taking into account partial agreement can increase the value of the coefficient of agreement. This is a typical result. Only if the cells with values of ω_{ij} greater than 0 and less than 1 are all empty, κ and κ_w will yield the same scores.

Table 1.3: **Partial Agreement Weights for Psychiatric Re-Diagnosis (data from Table 1.2)**

		Psychiatrist 2: Severity of Depression		
		1	2	3
Psychiatrist 1: Severity of Depression	1	1	.5	0
	2	.5	1	.5
	3	0	.5	1

When considering κ_w, researchers must take into account two issues. First, the rating scales must be at least at the ordinal scale level. If this is not the case, the magnitude of the discrepancy of ratings cannot be assessed. Second, there is some arbitrary component in the determination of the values and ratios of the weights, ω_{ij}. Therefore, great care must be taken not to manipulate results by optimizing the weights with the goal of maximizing (or minimizing) κ. Objective criteria such as pecuniary implications or severity of consequences from disagreement rarely exist that can be used to guide the selection of weights. Therefore, the choice of weights must always be made explicit.

1.3   Raw Agreement, Brennan and Prediger's κ_n, and a Comparison with Cohen's κ

The coefficient κ has met with critical appraisal because of a number of characteristics, the most problematic of which seems to be the one listed under (5) in Chapter 1.1. This characteristic indicates that Cohen's κ does not approximate the maximum value of $\kappa = 1$ if (1) the marginal totals are not uniformly distributed (cf. Feinstein & Cicchetti, 1990) while (2) at least one off-diagonal cell is non-zero. von Eye and Sörensen (1991) performed two sets of simulations to illustrate this effect. The first set simulates increasing agreement. The second set simulates increasing disagreement.

To start the simulations, the authors created a 2 x 2 cross-tabulation in which all cells had the frequency $m_{ij} = 1$. This arrangement comes with uniform marginal totals. Then, this same arrangement was altered in the two simulation runs. In the first run, in a series of 30 steps, the authors increased the frequency m_{11} by 3 per step. Thus, the sequence of frequencies 1, 4, 7, ..., 91 resulted for Cell 11. The other cells were held at $m_{ij} = 1$. The change of κ is depicted by the curve with the squares in Figure 1. Obviously, κ approaches an asymptote that is clearly below 1. In the present example, the asymptote is even below 0.5.

Figure 1 displays two comparison curves. The curve with the triangles describes the development of raw agreement, ra. An estimate of raw agreement can be calculated as

$$\hat{ra} = \frac{\sum_i m_{ii}}{N},$$

that is, the proportion of cases in the main diagonal, relative to the sample size. Figure 1, below, suggests that the asymptote for ra is 1.0. By increasing the frequencies in the main diagonal one can get as close to the asymptote as necessary. The coefficient can asymptotically reach 1 even if the marginals are extremely unevenly distributed. There is no significance test for the coefficient of raw agreement.

To solve the problem that the maximum degree of agreement is reduced when raters use the categories at different rates, Brennan and

Prediger (1981) propose substituting $\theta_2 = 1/g$ for the formulation used by Cohen, where g is the number of rating categories. This substitution leads to the definition of κ as

$$\kappa_n = \frac{\theta_1 - \dfrac{1}{g}}{1 - \dfrac{1}{g}}$$

An estimator of κ_n is then

$$\hat{\kappa}_n = \frac{\dfrac{\sum_i m_{ii}}{N} - \dfrac{1}{g}}{1 - \dfrac{1}{g}}.$$

To give an example, applying Brennan and Prediger's κ_n (1981) to the data in Table 1.2, one calculates

$$\hat{\kappa}_n = \frac{96/129 - 1/3}{1 - 1/3} = 0.616.$$

This value is greater than the $\kappa = 0.375$ estimated for the data in Table 1.2, but smaller than $ra = 0.744$. Notice that ra is the first term in the numerator of both κ and κ_n. That is, $ra = \theta_1$. When comparing κ and κ_n, one notices that the expected proportion of chance agreement (θ_2) changed from 0.591 to 0.333. This difference reflects the differences between the chance models. Whereas Brennan and Prediger's κ_n is based on a null model (no effects are assumed, not even main effects), Cohen's κ is based on the main effect model of rater independence (only differences in the frequencies are taken into account with which raters used rating categories). Chapters 2 and 3 provide more details on base models.

The second comparison curve in Figure 1, that with the diamonds, depicts the behavior of κ_n under the simulation conditions. The simulation results in Figure 1 suggest that

(1)   all three measures, κ, κ_n, and ra increase monotonically as the percentage of incidences of agreement increases;

(2)   all three measures approach an asymptote; this asymptote is 1 for both ra and κ_n, and it depends on the size of the table and the distribution of the marginals for κ;

(3)   as long as there are at least as many incidences of agreement as of

disagreement, the smallest possible value of the κ measures is zero, and the smallest value of *ra* is 0.5;

(4)   if $\kappa > 0$, $\kappa_n > 0$, and *ra* > 0.5, then *ra* > κ_n > κ.

In the second simulation run, the uniformly distributed 2 x 2 table was altered to illustrate the behavior of the three coefficients under the condition of increasing disagreement. Starting from the same 2 x 2 table with ones in all four cells, the frequency in the disagreement Cell 21 was increased by 3 in each of 30 steps. The results of this run are depicted in Figure 2.

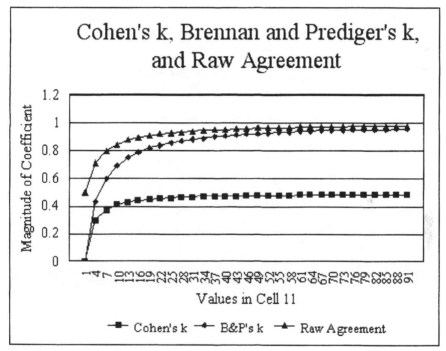

Figure 1: κ, κ_n, **and *ra* when agreement increases; marginals discrepant.**

The results in Figure 2 suggest that

(1)   Brennan and Prediger's κ_n and raw agreement decrease monotonically as disagreement increases; in contrast, Cohen's κ first decreases and then approximates zero.

(2)   all three measures have an asymptote. Raw agreement approximates zero; it is always positive; Brennan and Prediger's κ_n approximates -1, being always negative; and Cohen's κ

approximates zero, being always negative, but showing non-monotonic behavior;

(3)   if ra < 0.5, the three magnitudes can be ordered as follows: $ra > \kappa > \kappa_n$.

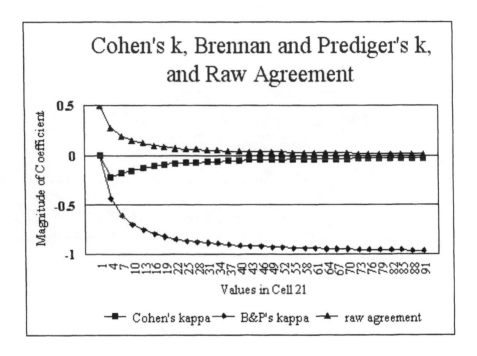

Figure 2: κ, κ_n, and *ra* when agreement decreases; marginals discrepant.

From the earlier considerations and these simulations, we conclude that

(1)   for ra > 0.5, which indicates that rater agreement is more likely than disagreement, the three measures ra, κ, and κ_n correlate strongly;

(2)   for ra > 0.5 and $\kappa \neq 1$, the magnitude of κ is only a weak indicator of strength of agreement; instead, κ indicates strength of agreement above and beyond the variation that can be explained by taking into account the main effects;

(3)   thus, except for the case in which $\kappa = 1.0$, κ is not a measure of raw agreement but a measure of agreement beyond chance;

(4)   researchers are well advised when they report raw agreement or Brennan and Prediger's κ_n in addition to Cohen's κ.

1.4   The Power of κ

In this section, power considerations for κ are reported for two cases. The first case covers sample size calculations for 2 x 2 tables. The second case is more general. It covers sample size calculations for tables of size 3 x 3 or larger for two or more raters.

The sample size requirements for κ under various hypotheses in 2 x 2 tables have been described by Cantor (1996). Based on Fleiss, Cohen, and Everitt (1969), the asymptotic variance of the estimate of κ can be given by Q/N, with

$$Q = (1 - \theta_2)^{-4} \left\{ \sum_i p_{ii}[(1 - \theta_2) - (p_{.i} + p_{i.})(1 - \theta_1)]^2 \right.$$
$$\left. + (1 - \theta_1)^2 \sum_i \sum_{i \neq j} p_{ij}(p_{.i} + p_{j.})^2 - (\theta_1\theta_2 - 2\theta_2 + \theta_1)^2 \right\},$$

where θ_1, θ_2, p_{ii}, $p_{i.}$, and $p_{.i}$, are defined as in Section 1.1, and p_{ij} indicates the probability of the off-diagonal cells, and p_j is the probability of Column j. Fortunately, the values of Q are tabulated for various values of $p_{i.}$ and $p_{.i}$ (Cantor, 1996, p. 152), so that hand calculations are unnecessary.

Now suppose, a researcher intends to test the null hypothesis H_0: $\kappa = \kappa_0$ with $\alpha = 0.05$ and power $1 - \beta = 0.80$. The sample size that is required for this situation is

$$N = \left[\frac{z_\alpha\sqrt{Q_0} + z_\beta\sqrt{Q_1}}{\kappa_1 - \kappa_0} \right]^2,$$

where z_α is the z-score that corresponds to the significance level α (e.g., for $\alpha = 0.05$, one obtains $z_{0.05} = 1.645$; accordingly, for $\beta = 0.2$, one obtains $z_{0.2} = 0.842$), Q_0 and Q_1 are the Q-scores for the null hypothesis and the alternative hypothesis, respectively. Note that the null hypothesis that $\kappa_0 = 0$ can be tested using this methodology. The values for Q can be either calculated or taken from Cantor's Table 1.

Consider the following example. A police officer and an insurance agent determine whether drivers in traffic accidents are at-fault or not-at-fault. A researcher intends to test the null hypothesis that $\kappa_0 = 0.3$ against the one-sided alternative hypothesis that $\kappa > 0.3$ with $\alpha = 0.05$ and power 0.8 for $\kappa_1 = 0.5$. We can take the two z-scores from above and find in the table $Q_0 = 0.91$ and $Q_1 = 0.75$. Inserting into the equation for N yields

$$N = \left[\frac{1.645\sqrt{0.91} + 0.842\sqrt{0.75}}{0.5 - 0.3} \right]^2 = 132.07.$$

Thus, to reject the null hypothesis that $\kappa_0 = 0.3$ in favor of the one-sided alternative hypothesis that $\kappa = 0.5$ with power 0.8 at a significance level of $\alpha = 0.05$, the researcher needs at least 132 traffic accidents in the sample.

For more hypothesis tests, including tests that compare rating patterns from two independent samples, see Cantor (1996). For tables larger than 2 x 2 see, for instance, Flack, Afifi, and Lachenbruch (1988).

A more general approach to power analysis for κ was recently proposed by Indurkhya, Zayas, and Buka (2004). The authors note that, under the usual multinomial sampling scheme, the cell frequencies follow a Dirichlet multinomial distribution. This distribution can then be used to estimate the probability that all raters choose category i. Based on this estimate, the authors derive a χ^2-distributed statistic for the null hypothesis that $\kappa = 0$ and an equation for the required sample size. This estimate depends on the probabilities that all raters chose a given rating category, the number of rating categories, the significance level, and the desired power. The authors present two tables with minimum required samples. The first table states the required sample sizes for the null hypothesis that $\kappa_0 = 0.4$ versus the alternative hypothesis that $\kappa_1 = 0.6$, for $\alpha = 0.05$ and $p = 0.8$. The second table presents the required sample sizes for the null hypothesis that $\kappa_0 = 0.6$ versus the alternative hypothesis that $\kappa_1 = 0.8$, for $\alpha = 0.05$ and $p = 0.8$. Table 1.4 summarizes these two tables.

Table 1.4:   **Minimum Required Sample Sizes for $\alpha = 0.05$ and $p = 0.8$ (adapted from Indurkhya et al., 2004)**

Null hypothesis: $\kappa_0 = 0.4$; alternative hypothesis: $\kappa_1 = 0.6$							
3 Categories			Number of raters				
π_1	π_2	π_3	2	3	4	5	6
0.1	0.1	0.8	205	113	83	68	59
0.1	0.4	0.5	127	69	50	40	35
0.33	0.33	0.34	107	58	42	35	30
							/ cont.

4 Categories				Number of raters				
π_1	π_2	π_3	π_4	2	3	4	5	6
0.1	0.1	0.1	0.7	102	42	38	32	29
0.1	0.3	0.3	0.3	88	30	30	29	27
0.25	0.25	0.25	0.25	60	28	27	25	25

Null hypothesis: $\kappa_0 = 0.6$; alternative hypothesis: $\kappa_1 = 0.8$

3 Categories			Number of raters				
π_1	π_2	π_3	2	3	4	5	6
0.1	0.1	0.8	172	102	77	66	58
0.1	0.4	0.5	102	60	46	40	35
0.33	0.33	0.34	87	52	39	33	30

4 Categories				Number of raters				
π_1	π_2	π_3	π_4	2	3	4	5	6
0.1	0.1	0.1	0.7	157	74	68	52	49
0.1	0.3	0.3	0.3	89	38	34	27	24
0.25	0.25	0.25	0.25	68	26	24	23	20

The sample sizes listed in Table 1.4 suggest that the required sample size decreases as the number of raters and the number of rating categories increase. In addition, as the probabilities of categories get more even, the required sample size increases. Donner and Eliasziw (1992) had presented similar results for the case of two raters and two rating categories.

1.5   Kendall's *W* for Ordinal Data

For ordinal (rank-ordered) data, Kendall's (1962) *W* is often preferred over κ (for interval level data, κ is equivalent to the well-known intraclass correlation; see Rae, 1988). W allows one to (1) compare many objects; (2) compare these objects in a number of criteria; and (3) take the ordinal nature of ranks into account. The measure W, also called *coefficient of concordance*, compares the agreement found between two or more raters with perfect agreement. The measure is

$$W = \frac{s}{\frac{1}{12} k^2 (N^3 - N)},$$

where N is the number of rated objects, k is the number of raters, and s is the sum of the squared deviations of the ranks R_i used by the raters from the average rank, that is,

$$s = \sum_i \left(R_i - \frac{\sum_i R_i}{N} \right)^2,$$

with $i = 1, ..., I$, the number of rating categories (i.e., the column sum). The maximum sum of squared deviations is

$$\frac{1}{12} k^2 (N^3 - N).$$

This is the sum s for perfect rater agreement.

For small samples, the critical values of W can be found in tables (e.g., in Siegel, 1956). For 8 or more objects, the χ^2-distributed statistic

$$X^2 = \frac{s}{\frac{1}{12} k(N^2 + N)} = k(N - 1)W$$

can be used under $df = N - 1$. Large, significant values of W suggest strong agreement among the k raters.

When there are ties, that is, judgements share the same rank, the maximum deviance from the average rank is smaller than the maximum deviance without ties. Therefore, a correction element is introduced in the denominator of the formula for Kendall's W. The formula becomes

$$W' = \frac{s}{\frac{1}{12} k^2 (N^3 - N) - k \sum_j (t_j^3 - t_j)},$$

where t_j is the number of tied ranks in the jth tie. This quantity is also called the *length of the jth tie*. If there are no ties, there will be N "ties" of length

1, and the second term in the denominator disappears. The corrected formula then becomes identical to the original formula.

Data example. The following example re-analyzes data presented by Lienert (1978). A sample of 10 participants processed a psychometric test. The solutions provided by the participants were scored according to the three criteria X = number of correct solutions, Y = number of correct solutions minus number of incorrect solutions, and Z = number of items attempted. The participants were ranked in each of these three criteria. We now ask how similar the rankings under the three criteria are. Table 1.5 displays the three series of ranks.

Table 1.5:   **Ranks of 10 Subjects in the Criteria X = Number of Correct Solutions, Y = Number of Correct Solutions minus Number of Incorrect Solutions, and Z = Number of Items Attempted**

	Participant									
Criterion	1	2	3	4	5	6	7	8	9	10
X	1	4.5	2	4.5	3	7.5	6	9	7.5	10
Y	2.5	1	2.5	4.5	4.5	8	9	6.5	10	6.5
Z	2	1	4.5	4.5	4.5	4.5	8	8	8	10
Sum	5.5	6.5	9	13.5	12	20	23	23.5	25.5	26.5

The average rank is calculated as the sum of all ranks over the number of participants. We obtain $\Sigma R = 165$ and $\overline{R} = 16.5$. For the sum of the squared deviations we obtain $s = (5.5 - 16.5)^2 + ... + (26.5 - 16.5)^2 = 591$. For the correction term, we calculate for X: $(2^3 - 2) + (2^3 - 2) = 12$; for Y: $(2^3 - 2) + (2^3 - 2) + (2^3 - 2) = 18$; and for Z: $(4^3 - 4) + (3^3 - 3) = 84$. The sum of these correction terms is 114. Inserting into the equation for W' yields

$$W' = \frac{591}{\frac{1}{12} 3^2(10^3 - 10) - 3 \cdot 114} = 0.828.$$

The value of $W' = 0.83$ suggests a high degree of concordance. That is, the three criteria suggest largely the same rankings. In the present example, this does not come as a surprise because there exists an algebraic relation between these three criteria. We find that $Y = X - F$ and $Z = X + F$, where F is the number of false solutions. Because of this dependency, the following significance test can be interpreted only as an illustration.

Inserting into the X^2 formula, we obtain $X^2 = 3(10 - 1)\ 0.828 = 22.349$. For $df = 9$, we find that $p = 0.0078$ and reject the null hypothesis of no concordance.

1.6 Measuring Agreement among Three or More Raters

The routine case of determining rater agreement involves two raters. However, occasionally three or more raters are used. In specific contexts, for example in political polls, large samples function as raters. The present section focuses on small numbers of raters. The formulas presented here describe measures for three raters. Generalizations to four or more raters are straightforward. When assessing the agreement among three raters, an $I \times I \times I$-table is created. That is, it is required again that all raters use the same rating categories. This table has three diagonals. The diagonal that contains the agreement cells is the one with like cell indexes, that is, iii. More specifically, the cells 111, 222, ..., III are the agreement cells.

For Cohen's non-weighted κ, we specify

$$\theta_1 = \sum_i p_{iii} \, ,$$

and

$$\theta_2 = \sum_{i=j=k} p_{i..}\, p_{.j.}\, p_{..k} \, ,$$

so that we obtain, as before,

$$\kappa = \frac{\theta_1 - \theta_2}{1 - \theta_2} \, .$$

An estimator of κ for three raters under multinomial sampling is then

$$\hat{\kappa} = \frac{N^2 \sum_i m_{iii} - \sum_i m_{i..}\, m_{.i.}\, m_{..i}}{N^3 - \sum_i m_{i..}\, m_{.i.}\, m_{..i}} \, .$$

The interpretation of κ for three or more raters is the same as for two raters.

For Brennan and Prediger's κ_n, we obtain the estimator

$$\hat{\kappa}_n = \frac{\dfrac{\sum_i m_{iii}}{N} - \dfrac{1}{g^2}}{1 - \dfrac{1}{g^2}}$$

For both, κ and κ_n for three or more raters, the binomial test can be used as significance test. Specifically, let p be estimated by θ_2 and $q = 1 - p$. The one-sided tail probability for $\kappa > 0$ is then

$$P = \sum_{j = \sum_i m_{iii}}^{N} \binom{N}{j} p^j q^{N-j}$$

The estimator of raw agreement among three raters is

$$\hat{ra} = \frac{\sum_i m_{iii}}{N}$$

Data example. For the following example, we analyze data from a study on the agreement of raters on the qualification of job applicants in a large agency in the United States.[2] A sample of 420 interview protocols was examined by three evaluators. Each evaluator indicated on a three-point scale the degree to which an applicant was close to the profile specified in the advertisement of the position, with 1 indicating very good match and 3 indicating lack of match. In the following paragraphs, we employ the coefficients just introduced. Table 1.6 displays the cross-classification of the three raters' judgements in tabular form. The table contains in its first column the cell indexes, in its second column the observed frequencies, followed by the expected frequencies that result for Cohen's κ, and the standardized residuals, $z_{iii} = \sqrt{\dfrac{(m_{iii} - \hat{m}_{iii})^2}{\hat{m}_{iii}}}$. The overall Pearson X^2 for this cross-classification is 723.26 ($df = 20$; $p < 0.01$), suggesting strong associations among the rater's judgements.

---

[2]Thanks go to Neal Schmitt for making these data available.

Table 1.6:   Agreement among Three Raters

Configuration	m	$\hat{m}$	z
111	61	7.401	19.701
112	15	9.287	1.875
113	1	12.638	-3.274
121	12	8.384	1.249
122	7	10.519	-1.085
123	5	14.316	-2.462
131	1	11.724	-3.132
132	4	14.711	-2.793
133	3	20.020	-3.804
211	10	9.167	.275
212	10	11.502	-.443
213	1	15.653	-3.704
221	14	10.384	1.122
222	36	13.029	6.364
223	16	17.731	-.411
231	5	14.521	-2.499
232	18	18.220	-.051
233	25	24.795	.041
311	1	11.951	-3.168
312	7	14.995	-2.065
313	7	20.407	-2.968
321	2	13.537	-3.136
322	18	16.985	.246
323	18	23.115	-1.064
331	0	18.931	-4.351
332	18	23.753	-1.180
333	105	32.326	12.782

For the three-dimensional version of Cohen's non-weighted κ, we calculate $\hat{\kappa} = 0.411$. For the three-dimensional variant of Brennan and Prediger's κ_n, we obtain $\hat{\kappa}_n = 0.416$. These values suggest that the three raters agreed over 40% more often than expected from either base model ($p < 0.01$ for both). For the coefficient of raw agreement, we obtain $\hat{ra} = 0.481$, suggesting that almost 50% of the decisions made by the three raters matched exactly.

This section covered the case in which researchers asks questions concerning unanimous agreement among three raters. Also interesting is the case in which some raters agree but not all. This case is covered in Section 2.4.1.

1.7   Many Raters or Many Comparison Objects

This section presents new applications of the coefficients discussed thus far in this text. There exist other coefficients that could be covered here, for example, a κ-statistic proposed by Fleiss (1981). However, we focus on applications of the statistics discussed thus far in this text.

Thus far in this book, methods and examples focused on the analysis of the agreement tables that can be created from crossing the judgements that two raters or observers provide for many objects. Consider the two psychiatrists in Section 1.1.1 who re-diagnosed a sample of 129 depressed patients. There are instances, however, in which either a large number of raters compares a small number of objects, or a large number of objects is compared in two characteristics. To give examples for the first case, over 200 million U.S. citizens compare two presidential candidates in every presidential election, millions of sports viewers compare the referees' calls with what they are presented in slow motion on TV, or students in one class compare the substitute teacher with the one they had before she fell sick. In this section, we discuss the analysis of data from this situation. To give examples for the second scenario, think of athletes that are compared with respect to their strength and their speed, or patients that are diagnosed twice, once before and once after some treatment.

The difference between these situations and the one we encounter in the rest of this text is that the cross-tabulation that is created is no longer a rater-by-rater table. Instead, it is either an object-by-object table (many objects are compared in one variable) or a variable-by-variable table (many objects are compared in two variables or twice in one variable; this applies accordingly when multiple variables are used). In the case of comparing two objects that are compared by many raters, this table results from crossing the ratings that one object received with the ratings that the other object received. Consider the case in which two objects, A and B, are rated using three rating categories. Then, the crossing of these categories yields a table as illustrated in Table 1.7.

Table 1.7:   Cross-Classification of the Judgements Given for Two Objects

		Object B Rating Categories		
		1	2	3
Object A Rating Categories	1	m_{11}	m_{12}	m_{13}
	2	m_{21}	m_{22}	m_{23}
	3	m_{31}	m_{32}	m_{33}

This table is parallel to the one given to illustrate the usual rater agreement table in Table 1.1. the diagonal cells, shaded, indicate the number of instances in which the two objects received the same ratings. The off-diagonal cells contain the instances in which the two objects received discrepant ratings.

The methods that can be used to analyze this type of table are the same as the methods that are used for the rater-by-rater tables. In the following data example, we cross the ratings that students received in two consecutive measurements. In a study by Finkelstein, von Eye, and Preece (1994), 114 adolescents were observed as to their physical pubertal development. The Tanner scales were used which indicate the progress is indicated that can be observed for an individual's development. The scale was truncated to have four scale points with 1 indicating pre-pubertal and 4 indicating physically mature. The first wave of measurements was made when the students were 10 years of age, the second wave was two years later. Table 1.8 displays the frequency table that results from crossing the ratings from the two observations.

Table 1.8: **Cross-Classification of Two Consecutive Ratings of Adolescents' Physical Pubertal Development**

	Time 2				
Time 1	1	2	3	4	Total
1	2	43	8	0	53
2	2	22	18	10	52
3	0	0	2	6	8
4	0	0	0	1	1
Total	4	65	28	17	114

From the row and column marginals, we see that, at Time 1, prepubertal and early pubertal ratings are far more frequent that ratings of advanced physical pubertal development. At Time 2, ratings of more advanced pubertal development increase in number. We now ask whether "ratings agree" over the two observation points, that is, whether development has taken place. In the present example, one expects "agreement" to be low. High agreement would indicate that no physical pubertal development takes place. Low or negative agreement would support the notion of development.

The Pearson X^2 for Table 1.8 is 49.95 ($df = 9; p < 0.01$), suggesting that the two measurements are strongly associated. However, this association is not carried by same ratings at both observation points. The estimate of Cohen's κ, -0.082, indicates that random guesses may be better than guesses based on the assumption of same ratings at both points in time. The difference is 8.2%. The estimate of the asymptotic standard error for this value is 0.042, $z = 1.952$, and $p(z) = 0.051$ (two-sided). We thus conclude that random guesses are almost significantly better than guesses based on the assumption of no development.

1.8   Exercises

1-1.   The following table contains an artificial 15-case by 3-variable data matrix. The 15 rows indicate 15 car models and the three columns of C1, C2, C3 indicate three car magazine editors' ratings on the car's comfort features: 1= Just About Average, 2 = Two Thumbs up. Present the data as a three-way configuration table as it appears in Table 1.6 of the text.

Cars	C1	C2	C3
1	1	1	1
2	1	1	2
3	1	2	2
4	1	1	1
5	2	2	2
6	1	1	1
7	2	1	1
8	2	2	2
9	1	2	2
10	1	1	1
11	1	2	1
12	2	1	1
13	1	1	1
14	2	2	2
15	1	2	1

1-2.   Estimate and interpret Cohen's κ for the agreement between editors C2 and C3.

1-3.   Estimate raw agreement and Brennan and Prediger's κ_n for the agreement between editors C2 and C3.

1-4.   Estimate the κ, κ_n, and ra for the agreement in all three editor pairs.

1-5.   Using the data in Table 1.6 of the text, create a 3 x 3 table between the first two raters and estimate κ, and weighted κ, using the weights of 1, 0.5, 0, 0.5, 1, 0.5, 0, 0.5, and 1.

1-6.   Using the table just created for question 1-5, calculate the conditional or partial κ estimates for all three categories.

1-7.   The following data are from a study by Jackson, Sher, Gotham, and Wood (2001) in which first-time college freshmen were classified into four groups based on their drinking pattern: 1 = Abstainer, 2 = Limited-effect Drinker, 3 = Moderate-effect Drinker, and 4 = Large-effect Drinker. Their drinking behavior was followed-up three years later and classified again. Calculate the proportion of college students whose drinking classification remained the same after three years. Estimate Cohen's κ and weighted κ_w between the classifications of Years 1 and 4. For the weighted κ_w, use $\omega = 1$ for the absolute agreement cells $(i = j)$, $\omega = 0.6667$ for cells $|i - j| = 1$, $\omega = 0.3333$ for cells $|i - j| = 2$, and $\omega = 0$ for cells $|i - j| = 3$. Are Cohen's κ and weighted κ_w significant at $\alpha = 0.05$? Also, calculate Pearson's X^2. Based on the three statistics, what would you say about the overlap between two classifications with a three-year interval?

	Three Years Later			
Freshmen	Abstainer (1)	Limited-effect Drinker (2)	Moderate-effect Drinker (3)	Large-effect Drinker (4)
1	35	14	11	2
2	4	14	17	3
3	5	31	41	25
4	10	2	56	171

2. Log-Linear Models of Rater Agreement

Measures such as κ, W, and the intraclass correlation coefficient are hugely popular, for good reasons. First, they are practically always applicable. Only in cases in which certain categories are not used at all, researchers have to resort to measures of raw agreement. Second, these coefficients condense important information in one coefficient that is easy to interpret. Correlation coefficients share this characteristic (see Chap. 4). Third, each of these coefficients is easy to calculate, and standard general purpose statistical software packages allow one to estimate these coefficients (mostly κ) and their standard errors.

However, κ has been reviewed critically for a number of reasons in addition to the ones listed under (2), (5) and (6) in Section 1.1.1 (Tanner, & Young, 1985). Specifically, issues of criticism include (a) the notion that there may be loss of information from summarizing characteristics of a table by a single measure and (b) the problem that values of κ from two or more tables cannot be compared. (Note that since this criticism, first solutions for this problem have been proposed; see Barnhart & Williamson, 2002; Cantor, 1996.) In addition, (c) unless κ approaches 1, the measure does not allow one to describe the structure of the joint distribution of raters' judgements. Therefore, modeling approaches have been marshaled (see, e.g., Agresti, 1988; Agresti, Ghosh, & Bini, 1995; Schuster & von Eye, 2001; Tanner & Young, 1985; von Eye & Schuster, 2000).

It is possible to mimic such coefficients as κ using log-multiplicative models (Schuster, 2001), under certain conditions. However, the motivation of this chapter is different. We present models that (1) allow one to test particular hypotheses that cannot be tested using a single coefficient, and (2) introduce hypotheses that capture some of the features of coefficients and then go beyond.

In the following chapter, we introduce readers to a series of log-linear models for rater agreement. We proceed in three steps. First, we introduce a *base model*. The following models of rater agreement are expressed in terms of deviations from this base model, more specifically, improvements over the base model. Second, we introduce a more *general manifest variable model of rater agreement*. This model contains all the terms and effects considered in this booklet. Third, we introduce a selection of *specific models*. These are models that can be derived from the general model by setting one or more parameters to zero. We begin in Chapter 2.1 with the base model.

2.1   A Log-Linear Base Model

For the following considerations, we use the design matrix approach to log-linear modeling. The design matrix approach is widely used in analysis of variance and regression analysis (e.g., Kirk, 1995; Neter, Kutner, Nachtsheim, & Wasserman, 1996; von Eye & Schuster, 1998b), and has also been employed in log-linear modeling (Christensen, 1997; Evers & Namboodiri, 1978; von Eye & Brandtstädter, 1998). Every log-linear model can be expressed using the design matrix approach. A brief introduction and examples are given in the following paragraphs and chapters.

For the following discussion of models, consider an I x J cross-classification. This table results from crossing the responses of Rater A with the responses of Rater B. This table is the *agreement table* that was introduced in Chapter 1. For the models discussed here, we require that $I = J$, that is, both raters use the same I rating categories. The base model that we consider is always

$$\log m = \lambda_0 + \lambda_i^A + \lambda_j^B + e,$$

where m_{ij} are the observed frequencies, λ_0 is the intercept parameter, λ_i^A are the main effect parameters for the row variable (Rater A), λ_j^B are the main effect parameters for the column variable (Rater B), and e_{ij} are the residuals. In the models that we present in the following chapters, rater agreement is compared with this base model and is parameterized in terms of deviations from this model.

Different base models are conceivable. For instance, Brennan and Prediger (1981; see Section 1.3, above) propose using a model in which the two terms, λ_i^A and λ_j^B are fixed to be zero. In the following sections, we enrich the base model given here by introducing various terms that allow one to consider characteristics of measurement models, or to test specific hypotheses.

The base model does not contain terms for the interaction between the two raters' responses. Interaction terms are not needed for the following two reasons. First, models for $I \times J$ cross-classifications that contain the A x B interaction are saturated. The present approach strives for more parsimonious models. Second, one reason why the raters' responses may be associated with each other is that they agree, but there may be other reasons for an association. The present approach attempts to model rater agreement.

However, before presenting the general model, we give an example of the design matrix approach to log-linear modeling (Christensen, 1997). Consider a 3 x 3 table. The log-linear base model for this table can be written in matrix form as

$$
\begin{bmatrix} \log m_{11} \\ \log m_{12} \\ \log m_{13} \\ \log m_{21} \\ \log m_{22} \\ \log m_{23} \\ \log m_{31} \\ \log m_{32} \\ \log m_{33} \end{bmatrix}
=
\begin{bmatrix}
1 & 1 & 0 & 1 & 0 \\
1 & 1 & 0 & 0 & 1 \\
1 & 1 & 0 & -1 & -1 \\
1 & 0 & 1 & 1 & 0 \\
1 & 0 & 1 & 0 & 1 \\
1 & 0 & 1 & -1 & -1 \\
1 & -1 & -1 & 1 & 0 \\
1 & -1 & -1 & 0 & 1 \\
1 & -1 & -1 & -1 & -1
\end{bmatrix}
\begin{bmatrix} \lambda_0 \\ \lambda_1^A \\ \lambda_2^A \\ \lambda_1^B \\ \lambda_2^B \end{bmatrix}
+
\begin{bmatrix} e_{11} \\ e_{12} \\ e_{13} \\ e_{21} \\ e_{22} \\ e_{23} \\ e_{31} \\ e_{32} \\ e_{33} \end{bmatrix},
$$

where the column vector on the left hand side of the equation contains the logarithms of the observed cell frequencies. The design matrix, X, on the right hand side of the equation, contains five column vectors. The first of these vectors contains only ones. It is the constant vector, used to estimate λ_0, the intercept parameter. The following two vectors represent the main effect of the first rater, A. The judgements from this rater appear in the rows of the 3 x 3 cross-classification. The first of these two vectors contrasts the first of the three categories with the third. The second of these vectors contrasts the second category with the third. The last two vectors of the design matrix represent the main effect of the second rater, B. The judgements from this rater appear in the columns of the 3 x 3 cross-classification. As for first rater, the first column main effect-vector contrasts the first with the third categories, and the second column main effect vector contrasts the second with the third categories. In different words, the first two main effect vectors contrast rows, whereas the second two main effect vectors contrast columns.

        To express the base model for the 3 x 3 example, we used the methods of effects coding. There exists a number of alternative coding schemes. Most prominent is dummy coding (see Christensen, 1997). The two methods of coding are equivalent in the sense that each model that can be expressed using one of the methods can be expressed equivalently using the other method. We select for the present context effects coding because this method makes it easy to show which cells are contrasted with each other.[3]

2.2   A Family of Log-Linear Models for Rater Agreement

Consider the I x I cross-classification of two raters' judgements of the same objects. In matrix notation, the base model given above can be expressed as $\log M = X\lambda + e$, where M is the column vector of observed frequencies, X is a design matrix (for an example see the matrix in Section 2.1, above), λ is a parameter vector, and e is the residual vector. For the models considered in the following chapters we use the form $X = [X_b, X_\delta, X_\beta, X_c]$, where X_b is the design matrix for the base model. An example was given in the last section. The adjoined, that is, horizontally merged, design matrices express those aspects of the bivariate frequency distribution that we consider when modeling rater agreement. X_δ is the design matrix that contains indicator variables for the cells that reflect rater agreement. These are typically the cells in the main diagonal of the I x I cross-classification. X_β is the design matrix that contains indicator variables used to specify

---

[3]Readers who use the SPSS package to recalculate the data examples in this booklet will notice that SPSS uses dummy coding by default.

characteristics of the measurement model concerning, for instance, the ordinal nature of the rating categories. X_c is the design matrix for covariate information. Accordingly, the parameter vector becomes $\lambda' = [\lambda'_b, \lambda'_\delta, \lambda'_\beta, \lambda'_c]$. The models presented in the following chapters use selections of the design matrices and parameter vectors. Any selection of these matrices is conceivable. Expressed in terms of the parameters that we estimate, the general model is

$$\log m = \lambda_0 + \lambda_i^A + \lambda_j^B + \delta + \beta u_i u_j + \lambda_{ij}^C + e.$$

The order of the terms on the right hand side of this equation is the same as in the matrix form of the equation. It should be noted, however, that the order of terms is arbitrary. It has no effect on the magnitude and standard errors of parameter estimates. These estimates can depend, however, on the other parameters in the model. The following sections discuss submodels and the meaning of parameters in more detail.

2.3 Specific Log-Linear Models for Rater Agreement

The following sections introduce readers to specific log-linear models for rater agreement. We begin with the equal weight agreement model, originally proposed by Tanner and Young (1985). For a discussion of such models in the context of symmetry and diagonal parameter models see Lawal (2001).

2.3.1 The Equal-Weight Agreement Model

The first model that we consider for rater agreement, adds one term to the base model introduced in Section 2.1. This model is

$$\log m = \lambda_0 + \lambda_i^A + \lambda_j^B + \delta + e,$$

where δ (delta) assigns weights to the cells in the main diagonal, that is, the cells where the two raters agree. Typically, one assigns equal weights to the cells in the main diagonal, that is,

$$\delta = \begin{cases} \delta & \textit{in diagonal cells} \\ 0 & \textit{otherwise.} \end{cases}$$

The resulting model is called *equal-weight agreement model* (Tanner & Young, 1985) or *diagonal set model* (Wickens, 1989). The model considers each rating category equally important for the assessment of rater agreement.

Data example. To illustrate the *equal weight agreement model*, we use data from a study by Lienert (1978), in which two teachers estimate the intelligence of 40 students by assigning them into four groups. The groups are 1: IQ < 90; 2: 90 ≤ IQ < 100; 3: 100 ≤ IQ < 110; and 4: IQ ≥ 110. Table 2.1 displays the cross-classification of the two teachers' ratings.

Table 2.1:   Cross-Classification of Two Teachers' Intelligence Ratings of Their Students

Intelligence Ratings		Teacher B				
		IQ < 90	90 - 99	100 - 109	IQ ≥ 110	Sum
T	IQ < 90	4	3	1	0	8
e						
a	90 - 99	1	5	2	2	10
c						
h	100 - 109	1	1	6	2	10
e						
r	IQ ≥ 110	0	1	5	6	12
A	Sum	6	10	14	10	40

$\hat{\kappa}$ for these data is 0.362 ($\hat{se}_{\kappa}$ = 0.106; z = 3.415; $p < 0.01$). We thus conclude that the two teachers agree in their intelligence ratings of their students 36.2% beyond chance, and that this degree of agreement is significantly greater than based on chance.

We now employ the *equal weight agreement model* described above. The explicit form for this model is, for the present 4 x 4 cross-classification,

$$
\begin{bmatrix}
\log m_{11} \\
\log m_{12} \\
\log m_{13} \\
\log m_{14} \\
\log m_{21} \\
\log m_{22} \\
\log m_{23} \\
\log m_{24} \\
\log m_{31} \\
\log m_{32} \\
\log m_{33} \\
\log m_{34} \\
\log m_{41} \\
\log m_{42} \\
\log m_{43} \\
\log m_{44}
\end{bmatrix}
=
\begin{bmatrix}
1 & 1 & 0 & 0 & 1 & 0 & 0 & 1 \\
1 & 1 & 0 & 0 & 0 & 1 & 0 & 0 \\
1 & 1 & 0 & 0 & 0 & 0 & 1 & 0 \\
1 & 1 & 0 & 0 & -1 & -1 & -1 & 0 \\
1 & 0 & 1 & 0 & 1 & 0 & 0 & 0 \\
1 & 0 & 1 & 0 & 0 & 1 & 0 & 1 \\
1 & 0 & 1 & 0 & 0 & 0 & 1 & 0 \\
1 & 0 & 1 & 0 & -1 & -1 & -1 & 0 \\
1 & 0 & 0 & 1 & 1 & 0 & 0 & 0 \\
1 & 0 & 0 & 1 & 0 & 1 & 0 & 0 \\
1 & 0 & 0 & 1 & 0 & 0 & 1 & 1 \\
1 & 0 & 0 & 1 & -1 & -1 & -1 & 0 \\
1 & -1 & -1 & -1 & 1 & 0 & 0 & 0 \\
1 & -1 & -1 & -1 & 0 & 1 & 0 & 0 \\
1 & -1 & -1 & -1 & 0 & 0 & 1 & 0 \\
1 & -1 & -1 & -1 & -1 & -1 & -1 & 1
\end{bmatrix}
\begin{bmatrix}
\lambda_0 \\
\lambda_1^A \\
\lambda_2^A \\
\lambda_3^A \\
\lambda_1^B \\
\lambda_2^B \\
\lambda_3^B \\
\delta
\end{bmatrix}
+
\begin{bmatrix}
e_{11} \\
e_{12} \\
e_{13} \\
e_{14} \\
e_{21} \\
e_{22} \\
e_{23} \\
e_{24} \\
e_{31} \\
e_{32} \\
e_{33} \\
e_{34} \\
e_{41} \\
e_{42} \\
e_{43} \\
e_{44}
\end{bmatrix}
$$

As in all log-linear models discussed here, the first column of the design matrix contains the constant vector. The following three columns represent the main effect of teacher A. In general, when a variable has c categories, the number of vectors needed to capture the main effect of this variable is $c - 1$. Accordingly, the next three columns represent the main effect of teacher B. The last column is specific to the present model. It posits that the weights in Cells 11, 22, 33, and 44 are the same. These are the cells that contain the students that obtained the same intelligence ratings from both teachers.

The log-linear model with the δ term describes the data well. Specifically, we calculate an overall goodness-of-fit likelihood ratio $X^2 = 10.08$ (LR-X^2). For $df = 8$, this value suggests no significant model-data discrepancies ($p = 0.259$). In addition, the parameter δ is significant ($\delta =$

1.22; $se_\delta = 0.33$; $z = 3.74$; $p < 0.01$). We thus conclude that this parameter makes a significant contribution to the explanation of the variability in this 4 x 4 cross-classification. The estimated expected frequencies for this model appear in Table 2.2.

Table 2.2: **Estimated Expected Cell Frequencies for Teachers' Intelligence Ratings Data (Equal Weight Agreement Model; for the observed cell frequencies, see Table 2.1)**

Intelligence Ratings		Teacher B				
		IQ < 90	90 - 99	100 - 109	IQ ≥ 110	Sum
T	IQ < 90	3.04	1.46	2.16	1.34	8
e						
a	90 - 99	0.96	5.29	2.32	1.43	10
c						
h	100 - 109	0.81	1.32	6.65	1.21	10
e						
r	IQ ≥ 110	1.19	1.93	2.87	6.02	12
A	Sum	6	10	14	10	40

The comparison of the observed with the expected cell frequencies indicates that the model-data fit is good overall. None of the standardized residuals, $(m_{ij} - \hat{m}_{ij})/\sqrt{\hat{m}_{ij}}$, is greater than the cutoff of 2.0, where $\hat{m}_{ij}$ is the estimated expected frequency of Cell ij.

For comparison, we also estimate the standard main effect model, that is, the model without the δ parameter. For this model, we obtain LR-X^2 = 23.79; $df = 9$, and $p = 0.0046$. This model is not good enough to explain the data. In addition, it is significantly worse than the equal weight agreement model ($\Delta X^2 = 13.71$; $\Delta df = 1$; $p < 0.01$). We thus retain the equal weight agreement model and conclude that placing equal weights on the main diagonal, that is, on the agreement cells, reflects the weights placed by the teachers on the rating categories. The two teachers do agree beyond chance.

In the present example, the κ and the log-linear analyses led us to the same conclusions. In both cases, we concluded that the raters agreed beyond chance. Concordance between these two approaches is certainly the routine result. However, there are instances in which the two approaches yield different results. Reasons for such differences include (1) model-data discrepancies in disagreement cells, that is, off-diagonal cells; (2) mis-specification of weights; and (3) skewed marginal distributions. In addition, the log-linear model may fail to describe the data properly when the observed frequencies are very large.

   From the perspective of the researcher, one may ask what to report in the presence of seemingly contradictory results. Beyond reporting both results, which is recommended, there is the option to decide in favor of interpreting κ and the option to decide in favor of interpreting the log-linear model. If the decision goes in favor of interpreting κ, emphasis is placed on the diagonal cells, whereas the distribution in the off-diagonal disagreement cells is given less importance. If, in contrast, the decision goes in favor of interpreting the log-linear model, emphasis is placed on the weights and their implications. Furthermore, and this is an option that comes only with the modeling approach, the model can be extended to accommodate additional hypotheses, for example, concerning covariates (see Sections 2.1 and 2.3.3).

Interpreting parameter δ in the equal weight agreement model. To illustrate the meaning of parameter δ in Tanner and Young's (1985) equal weight agreement model, consider the so-called *diagonal odds ratio* theta,

$$\theta = \frac{m_{ii}}{m_{ij}} \Big/ \frac{m_{ji}}{m_{jj}} = \frac{m_{ii} \, m_{jj}}{m_{ij} \, m_{ji}} ,$$

for $i \neq j$. This odds ratio relates the odds of finding a judgement in Cell ii and not in Cell ij to the odds of finding a judgement in Cell ji rather than in Cell jj. Now, replacing m_{ij} by the expression one would get in Tanner and Young's model, yields

$$\exp(2\delta) = \frac{m_{ii} \, m_{jj}}{m_{ij} \, m_{ji}} .$$

This expression shows that δ *can be interpreted as an indicator of the degree of agreement*. δ is related to the diagonal odds ratio by a simple, exponential transformation. More specifically, δ relates, just as does θ, the odds of finding a rating in Cell ii rather than in Cell ij to the odds of finding a rating in Cell ji rather than in Cell jj. The log-odds ratio is equal to 2δ. θ and $\exp(2\delta)$ are greater than 1 if the probability of finding ratings in the diagonal cells is greater than the probability of finding ratings in the off-diagonal cells.

2.3.2   The Weight-by-Response-Category Agreement Model

The Equal-Weight Agreement Model in Section 2.3.1 requires the assumption that agreement is equally important or carries equal weights across all categories. There may be research questions, however, where differential weights can be justified. Consider again the data example in Table 1.2. The different diagnoses come with different consequences. Patients diagnosed as clinically depressed will be admitted to the clinic. Patients diagnosed as not depressed will be sent home. The suffering caused by misdiagnoses, that is, false positives or false negatives, can be considerable. Therefore, researchers may consider a model that places weights on the three response categories such that, for instance, the "not depressed" category receives the lowest and the "clinically depressed" category the highest weight. Specifically, consider a model where

$$
\delta_{ij} = \begin{cases} \delta_i & \text{if } i = j \\ 0 & \text{otherwise} \end{cases}
$$

with, for example, $\delta_{11} = \delta_1$, $\delta_2 = 2\delta_1$, and $\delta_3 = 3\delta_1$. The selection of these weights and setting $\delta_1 = 1$, imply that the sixth column vector in the design matrix of the equal weight agreement model, that is, the vector $x_{6a}' = [1, 0, 0, 0, 1, 0, 0, 0, 1]$, is replaced by the vector $x_{6b}' = [1, 0, 0, 0, 2, 0, 0, 0, 3]$. Otherwise, this quasi-independence model is the same as the equal-weight model presented in Section 2.2.

Application of the weight-by-response-category agreement model to the depression diagnoses data in Table 1.2 yields LR-$X^2 = 13.49$ ($df = 3$; $p = 0.004$). Although this value indicates a significant improvement over the main effect model ($\Delta X^2 = 25.54$; $\Delta df = 1$; $p < 0.01$), the differential weight agreement model does not stand for itself; it is rejected. Furthermore, there is no indication that the differential weight agreement model is better than the model with equal weights. Table 2.3 displays the estimated expected cell frequencies for the equal weight agreement model and the differential weight agreement model (in *italics*).

Table 2.3:   **Estimated Expected Cell Frequencies for the Data in Table 1.2 for the Equal Weight Agreement Model and the Differential Weight Agreement Model (in *italics*)**

		Psychiatrist 2: Severity of Depression			Row Sums
		1	2	3	
Psychiatrist 1:	1	9.44	4.64	17.92	32
Severity of		*8.13*	*5.69*	*18.18*	
Depression	2	0.36	3.56	3.08	7
		0.73	*3.25*	*3.02*	
	3	2.19	4.81	83.00	90
		3.14	*4.07*	*82.79*	
Column Sums		12	13	104	N = 129

The comparison of these expected cell frequencies with the observed frequencies in Table 1.2 explains why the differential weight agreement model is not much better than the equal weight agreement model. The expected frequencies that were estimated for the differential weight agreement model are closer to the observed frequencies in five instances, whereas the expected frequencies estimated for the equal weight agreement model are closer in four instances.

2.3.3   Models with Covariates

The term *covariate* is often used "simply as an alternative name for explanatory variables ... that are likely to affect the response variable" (Everitt, 1998, p. 83). In the present context, a covariate is a categorical or a continuous variable that is likely to affect the joint frequency distribution of raters' judgements. In this section, we discuss two approaches to dealing with covariates. The first, proposed by Graham (1995) is concerned with categorical covariates. The second (von Eye & Schuster, 2000), is concerned with continuous covariates.

2.3.3.1 Models for Rater Agreement with Categorical Covariates

Consider a study in which two raters evaluate a sample of students, half of which are female and half of which are male. The usual aggregated-over-strata analysis using Cohen's κ or one of the log-linear models proposed in the literature does not allow one to discuss the effect of sex on agreement. One option would be to analyze the two strata separately and then compare the two κ values or the parameters estimated for the two samples. Another option, proposed by Graham (1995), involves extending Tanner and Young's (1985) model such that it incorporates covariates.

Consider again the Tanner and Young model which is

$$\log m = \lambda_0 + \lambda_i^A + \lambda_j^B + \delta + e,$$

where δ assigns weights to the cells in the main diagonal, that is, the cells where the two raters agree. To illustrate this model, we use a 2 x 2 cross-classification, that is, the simplest possible case in which two raters use only two categories for their judgements. This cross-classification appears in Table 2.4.

Table 2.4:   2 x 2 Cross-Classification of Two Raters' Judgements

		Rater B Rating Categories	
		1	2
Rater A Rating Categories	1	m_{11}	m_{12}
	2	m_{21}	m_{22}

Suppose that Table 2.4 describes the case in which two strata were aggregated and the entire sample is analyzed as one group. For the model proposed by Graham (1995), we now decompose the arrangement in Table 2.4 to accommodate the two strata. We obtain Table 2.5.

The 2 x 2 x 2 cross-classification in Table 2.5 contains two subtables, one for each of the two strata. The subscripts denote the stratum, the rating categories of Rater A, and the rating categories of Rater B, in that order. The log-linear model proposed by Graham (1995) to assess the agreement between Rater A and Rater B in the two strata is

$$\log m = \lambda_0 + \lambda_i^A + \lambda_j^B + \lambda_k^S + \delta^{AB} +$$
$$\lambda_{ik}^{AS} + \lambda_{jk}^{BS} + \delta_k^{ABS} + e,$$

where A and B denotes the two raters, S denotes the strata, and i, j, and k index Rater A, Rater B, and the strata. Double-subscripted terms indicate interactions. More specifically, double-subscripted terms represent partial associations between the superscripted variables, controlling for the variables not listed in the superscript (more detail follows). The terms in the first line of this equation are the same as for the Tanner and Young model in Section 2.3.1. The terms in the second line are new to Graham's extended covariate model.

Table 2.5: **2 x 2 Cross-Classification of Two Raters' Judgements in Two Strata**

Stratum 1		Rater B Rating Categories		Stratum 2		Rater B Rating Categories	
		1	2			1	2
Rater A Rating Categories	1	m_{111}	m_{112}	Rater A Rating Categories	1	m_{211}	m_{212}
	2	m_{121}	m_{122}		2	m_{221}	m_{222}

The first of the double-subscripted λ-terms, λ_{ik}^{AS}, is the partial association between Rater A and the stratum variable, controlling for Rater B. In different words, this parameter indicates the degree to which the judgements of Rater A vary across the strata. In a parallel fashion, the second double-subscripted term, λ_{jk}^{BS}, indicates the degree to which the judgements of Rater B vary across the strata. This partial association controls for Rater A.

The parameter δ^{AB} is identical to the δ parameter in Section 2.3.1. The stratum variable is controlled for. That is, a variation across the strata is not assumed. In contrast, the parameter δ_k^{ABS} does vary across the strata. There are as many parameters δ_k^{ABS} as there are strata, that is, this parameter is stratum-specific.

Identifiability. It is important to realize that the one-covariate model for the 2 x 2 x 2 cross-classification in Table 2.5 is over-saturated. There is no degree of freedom left for statistical testing. In fact, the degrees of freedom for this model are $df = -1$, if we place no constraints. More specifically, there are eight cells in the cross-tabulation. Four degrees of freedom are needed to model the intercept parameter, λ_0, and the three main effect parameters. Two more degrees of freedom are needed for the partial associations of the raters with the two-category stratum variable, and one degree of freedom for the double-subscripted δ parameter. For the triple-superscripted δ parameter we need two more degrees of freedom (one for each stratum). The sum of these is $df = -1$. Thus, we need to find a way to make this model identifiable.

There are several ways to deal with the problem of an over-saturated model. The first and most obvious is to use more rating categories and/or more strata than just two. This, however, may not always be possible, in particular when the number of strata is naturally constrained to two as in the case of male and female. Two constraints are typically considered. First, one can set either the parameter $\delta_{k=1}^{ABS} = 0$ or $\delta_{k=2}^{ABS} = 0$. The stratum for which the parameter is set to zero then serves as a reference category. This constraint reduces the number of stratum-specific parameters that are estimated by one. The model degrees of freedom are then zero. This model is saturated, but the parameters can be estimated and interpreted. The second option is to set $\sum_k \delta_k^{ABS} = 0$. This would be equivalent to the zero sum constraint that is in place for the main effect parameters. This second option also reduces the number of parameters by one. In general, both of these options reduce the number of parameters by one, regardless of the number of strata. The design matrix for the two-strata equal weight agreement model with the constraint that $\delta_{k=2}^{ABS} = 0$ is

$$
X = \begin{bmatrix}
1 & 1 & 1 & 1 & 1 & 1 & 1 & 1 \\
1 & 1 & 1 & -1 & 1 & -1 & 0 & 0 \\
1 & 1 & -1 & 1 & -1 & 1 & 0 & 0 \\
1 & 1 & -1 & -1 & -1 & -1 & 1 & 1 \\
1 & -1 & 1 & 1 & -1 & -1 & 1 & 0 \\
1 & -1 & 1 & -1 & -1 & 1 & 0 & 0 \\
1 & -1 & -1 & 1 & 1 & -1 & 0 & 0 \\
1 & -1 & -1 & -1 & 1 & 1 & 1 & 0
\end{bmatrix}.
$$

As always, the first column in this matrix is the constant vector. The following three columns represent the main effects of the three variables S, A, and B. The fifth vector in X represents the interaction between Rater A and the grouping variable, S. The vector results from multiplying the corresponding elements of the vectors for A and S with each other. The sixth vector represents the interaction between rater B and the grouping variable. It results from multiplying the corresponding elements of vectors B and S with each other. The second last vector represents the double-superscripted term, δ^{AB}. Using this term, it is proposed that Raters A and B agree when the data are aggregated over the two strata. In the last vector, it is proposed that the agreement in Stratum 1 differs from the agreement in Stratum 2.

Data example. For the following example we use data from a study by von Eye, Jacobson, and Wills (1990). In this study, 182 individuals, 133 of which were female, rated a number of proverbs as to the concreteness of their meaning. The proverbs were rated as either abstract (1) or concrete (2). The following analyses use the ratings of the first two proverbs. The stratification variable is Gender, coded as 1 = female and 2 = male. Table 2.6 displays the observed frequency distribution for the two proverbs.

Table 2.6:   **Observed Frequency Distribution of the 2 (Gender) x 2 (Proverb 1) x 2 (Proverb 2) Cross-Classification**

Females		Proverb 2		Males		Proverb 2	
		1	2			1	2
Proverb 1	1	20	23	Proverb 1	1	12	6
	2	8	82		2	6	25

Raw agreement in this table is 76.37% overall, and 76.69% in the female group, and 75.51% in the male group. We now ask whether an equal weight agreement model with Gender as covariate allows us to provide a more detailed picture of the observed frequency distribution. We estimate four hierarchically related models:

(1)   the main effect model $\log m = \lambda_0 + \lambda_i^G + \lambda_j^{P1} + \lambda_k^{P2} + e$,

(2)   the equal weight agreement model without the triple-superscripted association term, that is,

$$\log m = \lambda_0 + \lambda_i^G + \lambda_j^{P1} + \lambda_k^{P2} + \delta^{P1,P2} + \lambda_{ij}^{G,P1} + \lambda_{ik}^{G,P2} + e,$$

which states that the agreement concerning the two proverbs can be explained from the assumption that agreement is the same in both gender groups; and

(3)   the equal weight agreement model including the triple-superscripted association term, that is,

$$\log m = \lambda_0 + \lambda_i^G + \lambda_j^{P1} + \lambda_k^{P2} + \delta^{P1,P2} + \lambda_{ij}^{G,P1} + \lambda_{ik}^{G,P2} + \delta_k^{G,P1,P2} + e,$$

which states that the agreement in the female group differs from that in the male group. The vector used for the triple-superscripted term, $\delta_k^{G,P1,P2}$, is $X_7' = [1, 0, 0, 1, 0, 0, 0, 0]$.

(4)   In addition, we estimate a model that is hierarchically related to Models 1 and 3 but not to Model 2. This is the model that only uses the triple subscripted δ term, thus proposing that there is no common agreement structure but only a gender-specific structure. This model only uses the triple-superscripted δ term but not the

double-subscripted one. It is the model

$$\log m = \lambda_0 + \lambda_i^G + \lambda_j^{P1} + \lambda_k^{P2} +$$
$$\lambda_{ij}^{G,P1} + \lambda_{ik}^{G,P2} + \delta_k^{G,P1,P2} + e.$$

Table 2.7 gives an overview of the goodness-of-fit results and compares the models where possible.

Table 2.7: Four Models of the Agreement on the Concreteness of Two Proverbs

Model	$LR\text{-}X^2$	df	p	ΔX^2 to Model 1; Δdf; p	ΔX^2 to Model 2; Δdf; p
(1)	39.32	4	< 0.01	-	
(2)	0.01	1	0.94	39.31; 3; < 0.01	-
(3)	0.00	0	-	39.32; 4; < 0.01	0.01; 1; 0.92
(4)	11.06	1	< 0.01	28.26; 3; < 0.01	-

The results in Table 2.7 suggest that the main effect model (Model 1) is not tenable, and neither is the model that includes only the triple subscripted term, Model 4. Model 4 does provide a significant improvement over Model 1. However, because it is not tenable by itself, we cannot interpret the parameters. The two models that include the double-subscripted parameter, Models 2 and 3, are both tenable and significantly better than Model 1. In addition, they do not differ signficantly from each other, because the $LR\text{-}X^2$ for Model 2 is close to zero. Because Model 2 is more parsimonious than Model 3, we retain Model 2.

The interpretation of these results can first focus on the fact that the triple-superscripted term, $\delta_k^{P1,P2,G}$, is not needed. In fact, the z-score for this parameter in the saturated Model 3 is 0.08. This result suggests that the agreement pattern is not gender-specific. Thus, this parameter is not needed. In concordance with this result, the z-score for the parameter $\delta^{P1,P2}$ is 4.55 ($p < 0.01$), suggesting that the hypothesis of gender-unspecific agreement patterns allows one to explain a significant portion of the frequency distribution. This explanation can be based on the equal weight hypothesis.

Extensions. A natural extension of the above model was proposed already by Graham (1995). This extension involves two or more covariates. A second extension that has not been discussed in the literature involves the grouping of strata, if more than two strata are studied. It is possible to specify hypotheses such that for some strata agreement structures are proposed that differ from the agreement structures for other groups of strata or individual strata. A third extension involves differential weight agreement models that assign different weights to the agreement cells in the main diagonal(s) (see Section 2.3.2).

2.3.3.2 Models for Rater Agreement with Continuous Covariates

In many instances, covariates are continuous rather than categorical, and many researchers are reluctant to categorize continuous information. To give three examples, (1) intelligence may be considered a covariate of ratings on performance in English, (2) verbosity has been used as a covariate to explain raters' evaluations of interpretations of proverbs (von Eye & Schuster, 2000), and (3) the number of leisure activities has been used as a covariate in the evaluation of performance in spatial-visual performance (Glück & von Eye, 2000). To be able to accommodate continuous covariates, von Eye and Schuster (2000) proposed extending the equal weight agreement model by a term that contains the covariate. Consider again the general model presented in Section 2.2,

$$\log m = \lambda_0 + \lambda_i^A + \lambda_j^B + \delta + \beta u_i u_j + \lambda^C + e.$$

By setting $\beta u_i u_j = 0$, we obtain an equal weight agreement model (δ = constant) or a differential weight agreement model (δ not constant) with one covariate, C. The covariate is typically a single score that characterizes all individuals in a cell. Examples of such scores include the mean, the median, the variance, and the mode. Frequencies and probabilities have also been used. λ^C is the weight that the covariate has for the explanation of the observed frequency distribution. Thus, the model with one covariate is

$$\log m = \lambda_0 + \lambda_i^A + \lambda_j^B + \delta + \lambda^C + e.$$

Using this model, researchers propose that above and beyond the contributions made by the main effects and the δ parameter, there is a covariate that allows one to make a significant contribution to the explanation of the joint frequency distribution of two raters' judgements. It is important to note that this model does not include the associations between the raters' main effects and the covariate, even though these associations may be worth considering.

To illustrate this model, consider a 3 x 3 cross-classification that is analyzed under the hypothesis of an equal weight agreement model using one additional covariate. Rater A's ratings are given in the rows, Rater B's ratings are given in the columns. To simplify presentation, we present all columns in a single design matrix and a single parameter vector. The resulting complete model appears in the following equation.

$$
\begin{bmatrix} \log m_{11} \\ \log m_{12} \\ \log m_{13} \\ \log m_{21} \\ \log m_{22} \\ \log m_{23} \\ \log m_{31} \\ \log m_{32} \\ \log m_{33} \end{bmatrix} =
\begin{bmatrix}
1 & 1 & 0 & 1 & 0 & 1 & c_{11} \\
1 & 1 & 0 & 0 & 1 & 0 & c_{12} \\
1 & 1 & 0 & -1 & -1 & 0 & c_{13} \\
1 & 0 & 1 & 1 & 0 & 0 & c_{21} \\
1 & 0 & 1 & 0 & 1 & 1 & c_{22} \\
1 & 0 & 1 & -1 & -1 & 0 & c_{23} \\
1 & -1 & -1 & 1 & 0 & 0 & c_{31} \\
1 & -1 & -1 & 0 & 1 & 0 & c_{32} \\
1 & -1 & -1 & -1 & -1 & 1 & c_{33}
\end{bmatrix}
\begin{bmatrix} \lambda_0 \\ \lambda_1^A \\ \lambda_2^A \\ \lambda_1^B \\ \lambda_2^B \\ \delta \\ \lambda^C \end{bmatrix} +
\begin{bmatrix} e_{11} \\ e_{12} \\ e_{13} \\ e_{21} \\ e_{22} \\ e_{23} \\ e_{31} \\ e_{32} \\ e_{33} \end{bmatrix}
$$

In the design matrix, the four columns after the constant represent the main effects of the rows and the columns. The second last vector represents the equal weight agreement hypothesis known from Section 2.3.1. The last vector in X contains the scores of the covariate. For each of the column vectors in X, one parameter is estimated. These parameters appear in the vector that is pre-multiplied by the design matrix, X.

Data example. To illustrate the equal weight agreement model with covariate, we use data from the clinical study that yielded the data in Table 1.2, above. In this study, two psychiatrists evaluated the severity of the patients' depression using the rating categories 1 = not depressed, 2 = mildly depressed, and 3 = clinically depressed. We now use the variable severity of paranoia as a covariate in the analysis of rater agreement and ask whether knowledge about the psychiatrists' ratings of paranoia in the same patients allows us to explain the agreement pattern concerning the severity of these patients' depression. von Eye and Schuster (2000) had shown that the hypothesis of equal weight agreement does not enable one to explain the data in Table 1.2.

The two psychiatrists evaluated the patients' files also on a severity of paranoia scale with 1 = not paranoid, 2 = intermediate, and 3 = paranoid. The rater agreement/disagreement frequencies in the nine cells of the 3 x 3 cross-classification of the paranoia ratings of the two raters are $c_{ij}' = [17, 27, 3, 16, 45, 14, 1, 3, 3]$ (these data will be used again in Section 3.2). Table 2.8 displays the observed frequencies from Table 1.2 along with the expected cell frequencies (in *italics*), estimated under the equal weight agreement model with the joint ratings of paranoia as a covariate. The model is

$$\log m = \lambda_0 + \lambda_i^A + \lambda_j^B + \delta + \lambda^C + e.$$

Table 2.8: **Two Raters' Perception of Severity of Depression; Equal Weight Agreement Model with Covariate (observed and *expected* cell frequencies)**

		Severity of Depression			Row Sums
		1	2	3	
Severity of Depression	1	11 *11.23*	2 *1.53*	19 *19.23*	32
	2	1 *0.35*	3 *3.33*	3 *3.33*	7
	3	0 *0.42*	8 *8.14*	82 *81.44*	90
Column Sums		12	13	104	N = 129

The overall goodness-of-fit for this model is excellent. Table 2.9 displays the goodness-of-fit results for the three comparison models

(1)   main effect base model
$$\log m = \lambda_0 + \lambda_i^A + \lambda_j^B + e,$$

(2)   equal weight agreement model without covariate

$$\log m = \lambda_0 + \lambda_i^A + \lambda_j^B + \delta + e,$$

and

(3)   equal weight agreement model with covariate (see above).

The results in Table 2.9 suggest that neither the main effect model (1) nor the plain equal weight agreement model (2) are tenable, although the equal weight agreement model comes with a significant improvement over the main effect model. Including the covariate changes the picture significantly. The equal weight agreement model plus covariate is a significant improvement over both other models, and is tenable by itself. We thus conclude that we are able to explain the agreement pattern of the two psychiatrists based on an equal weight agreement hypothesis if we take into account the paranoia ratings of the two psychiatrists.

Table 2.9:   **Goodness-of-Fit Results for Psychiatric Diagnosis Data in Tables 2.2 and 3.9 under Three Log-Linear Models**

Model	$LR\text{-}X^2$	df	p	ΔX^2 to Model 1; Δdf; p	ΔX^2 to Model 2; Δdf; p
(1)	39.03	4	< 0.01	-	
(2)	9.22	3	0.03	29.81; 1; < 0.01	-
(3)	1.85	2	0.40	37.18; 2; < 0.01	7.37; 1; < 0.01

When looking at the parameters of this model, we find that the two interesting parameters, δ and λ^C are both significant. The estimate for the equal weight agreement parameter δ is -0.16 with a standard error of $se_\delta = 0.074$, $z = -2.20$, and $p = 0.0139$. The estimate for λ^C is 3.65 with a standard error of $se_\lambda = 1.13$, $z = 3.23$, and $p < 0.01$. We thus conclude that

(1)   the joint frequency distribution of the ratings of the two psychiatrists is not random. This conclusion can be drawn from the rejection of the main effect model (see Table 3.10). There must be an association between the ratings.

(2)   This association cannot be explained solely on the basis of the equal weight agreement hypothesis. Although this hypothesis does allow us to significantly improve the data description (see Table

3.10), the model is not good enough to stand by itself.

(3)   Taking into account the knowledge about the same raters'
        evaluations of the paranoid elements in the patients' depression in
        the form of a covariate improves the model fit dramatically and
        significantly. In this *equal weight agreement model with one
        covariate*, both interesting parameters, δ and λ^c, are significant,
        thus explaining significant portions of the deviation from the base
        model of variable main effects.

Caveat. The present approach is attractive because it only requires a minor
extension of Tanner and Young's (1985) equal weight agreement model.
Parameter interpretation, however, may be inconclusive. The parameters
are related to the design matrix and the observed cell frequencies by
$\lambda = (X'X)^{-1}X'\log m$, where the prime symbol indicates that the design
matrix was transposed, and $^{-1}$ indicates inversion. The parameters can only
be interpreted as solely reflecting the effects specified in the columns of X
if these columns are orthogonal for single parameters or block-orthogonal
for groups of parameters such as all parameters that reflect the same main
effect or interaction. In addition, the inverse $(X'X)^{-1}$ must exist. Parameters
are still interpretable if the effects can be expressed in terms of odds ratios
(von Eye & Brandtstädter, 1998). However, extending the model by adding
a vector of observed frequencies as in the last example, may cause
problems for parameter interpretation because this vector is bound to be
correlated with other vectors in the design matrix.

        Three methods to interpret and assess the contribution of the
covariate have been discussed. The first method involves estimating a
hierarchy of models in a fashion analogous to hierarchical regression. In the
above example, we created such a hierarchy by first estimating the main
effect model as the base model. Then, we estimated the plain equal weight
agreement model. This model is hierarchically related to the main effect
model because it contains one additional parameter while including all
parameters of the main effect model. The equal weight agreement model
with covariate is hierarchically related to the one without covariate,
because it contains one additional parameter and keeps all other parameters.
Therefore, the gain in model fit must be caused by the additional
information in the design matrix, and this information is the covariate
vector.

        The second method involves centering the covariate, a procedure
that is said to reduce the correlations with other column vectors in the

design matrix. However, unless the conditions found in the discussion provided by von Eye and Schuster (1998b) are met, centering rarely has the desired effect.

The third method involves considering the interpretation of the covariate parameter itself.[4] Consider the logarithm of the expected frequency in Cell ij, that is, $\log(\hat{m}_{ij})$. The difference of this score from the same expected frequency augmented by one unit of the covariate yields

$$\log(\hat{m}_{ij} + 1) - \log(\hat{m}_{ij}) = \lambda^C .$$

We thus obtain

$$\lambda^C = \log\left(\frac{\hat{m}_{ij} + 1}{\hat{m}_{ij}}\right),$$

that is, the *logit* which indicates the change in the probability of Cell ij when the score of the covariate changes by one unit.

Extensions. Two natural extensions of the equal weight agreement model with one covariate are the model with differential weights (see Section 2.3.2) and the model with multiple covariates. The former model has the same form as the equal weight model. The two models differ only in the entries of the weight vector. The latter model can be written as

$$\log m = X^b\lambda^b + \delta + X^c\lambda^c + e,$$

where X^b is the design matrix for the base model, λ^b is the parameter vector for the base model, X^c is matrix with covariate scores in its columns, and λ^C is the parameter vector for the covariates. Another extension could be a model in which a categorical covariate is treated as proposed by Graham (1995; see Section 2.3.3.1) and, simultaneously, one or more continuous covariates are treated as discussed in the present section. A special application of covariate models to rater-specific trends is presented in Section 2.4.2.

---

[4] The following explanation was provided by Christof Schuster. Our thanks go to him for this contribution.

2.3.4   Rater Agreement plus Linear-by-Linear Association for Ordinal Variables

Thus far, we have used a base model that presupposes that the rating categories are scaled at the nominal level. In many instances, however, rating categories are at the ordinal, interval, or even ratio scale levels. For instance, grades in school are at the ordinal level, the scores in Olympic figure skating are at the ordinal level, and the speed measured by police speed traps may even be at the interval level. If rating categories are at scale levels higher than the nominal level, the cross-classification of two raters' evaluations can carry information that is neither used by the original coefficient κ nor by the log-linear models employed thus far. Therefore, Agresti (1988) proposed *models of baseline association plus agreement for ordinal or higher level rating variables*. For the present purposes, we consider models of the form

$$\log m = \lambda_0 + \lambda_i^A + \lambda_j^B + \beta u_i u_j + \delta + e,$$

where the $u_1 < ... < u_I$ are fixed or known scores of the rating categories, typically their ranks (natural numbers: 1, 2, 3, ...), β (beta) is a weight parameter, and I is the number of rating categories. This model contains no covariates, that is, $\lambda^C = 0$. However, covariates can be considered (see Section 2.3.5, below). The weights in the main diagonal can be treated as before, that is, as either equal or differential. Because there is only one β, a model with these specifications requires only one parameter in addition to the parameters required by the equal weight agreement model discussed in Section 2.3.1.

There is a number of ways to define the u scores. If, for instance, the intervals between the response categories are equal as they are when $u_i = i$, with $i = 1, ..., I$, the measurement model represents the uniform linear-by-linear association model proposed by Goodman (1979). The scores for the response categories can also refer to (a) the midpoint of the ordinal scale, for example, the midpoint of the grade scales used in schools; (b) the mean of some continuous scale from which the categories have been derived by way of categorization; or (c) integer scores. Most typically, researchers use the ranks themselves for scores, that is $u_i = i$ and $u_j = j$, for $i, j = 1, ..., I$ (cf. Clogg, & Shihadeh, 1994). Each of these choices completely specifies the distances between categories.

The multiplication of u-scores with each other indicates that taking into account the ordinal nature of variables implies including an interaction term in the agreement model. This interaction term involves only one parameter, β. The interaction itself is defined by the element-wise multiplication of the rank scores used by the two raters. This specification of an interaction can be viewed parallel to the ones used in regression and analysis of variance. The local log-odds ratios for this model, given in Agresti (1988) all have the same sign. If the above model is specified without the δ term, it is equivalent to the uniform association model (Goodman, 1979).

Without the δ term, the model given above describes some form of association between two raters' responses. Including the δ term implies a focus on those cells that contain the frequencies with which the two raters provide the same score for an object. The equal weight agreement model with linear-by-linear interaction thus decomposes two raters' responses into three parts. The first is that explained by chance, that is, the proposition that the two raters are independent. This part is specified in the main-effects-only base model. The second part is that of baseline association, represented by the $\beta u_i u_j$ term, and the third part is that element of agreement that goes beyond the first two parts and reflects the raters' using identical ratings. This last part is represented by the δ term.

To illustrate the model $\log m = \lambda_0 + \lambda_i^A + \lambda_j^B + \beta u_i u_j + \delta + e$, we use a 3 x 3 cross-tabulation in which the judgements of Rater A are arranged in the rows and the judgements of Rater B are arranged in the columns. The explicit form of this model is

$$
\begin{bmatrix}
\log m_{11} \\
\log m_{12} \\
\log m_{13} \\
\log m_{21} \\
\log m_{22} \\
\log m_{23} \\
\log m_{31} \\
\log m_{32} \\
\log m_{33}
\end{bmatrix}
=
\begin{bmatrix}
1 & 1 & 0 & 1 & 0 & 1 & 1 \\
1 & 1 & 0 & 0 & 1 & 2 & 0 \\
1 & 1 & 0 & -1 & -1 & 3 & 0 \\
1 & 0 & 1 & 1 & 0 & 2 & 0 \\
1 & 0 & 1 & 0 & 1 & 4 & 1 \\
1 & 0 & 1 & -1 & -1 & 6 & 0 \\
1 & -1 & -1 & 1 & 0 & 3 & 0 \\
1 & -1 & -1 & 0 & 1 & 6 & 0 \\
1 & -1 & -1 & -1 & -1 & 9 & 1
\end{bmatrix}
\begin{bmatrix}
\lambda_0 \\
\lambda_1^A \\
\lambda_2^A \\
\lambda_1^B \\
\lambda_2^B \\
\beta \\
\delta
\end{bmatrix}
+
\begin{bmatrix}
e_{11} \\
e_{12} \\
e_{13} \\
e_{21} \\
e_{22} \\
e_{23} \\
e_{31} \\
e_{32} \\
e_{33}
\end{bmatrix}
$$

The first five columns of this design matrix contain the constant vector and the two main effect vectors each for the two raters. The sixth column contains the vector for the $\beta u_i u_j$ term, that is, the linear-by-linear interaction. The entries in this vector are created by multiplying the cell indices with each other. For example, the indices of the first cell are 1 and 1. Thus, the entry for Cell 11 is $1 \cdot 1 = 1$. Accordingly, the entry for Cell 23 is $2 \cdot 3 = 6$, and so forth. The seventh vector contains the vector for the equal weight agreement hypothesis. We know this vector from the earlier examples.

Data example. For the following empirical example, we use data published by Bortz, Lienert, and Boehnke (1990). The example involves a larger cross-classification than the above 3 x 3. However, the design matrix can be created accordingly, using the same concepts. The authors report about a study in which two TV journalists, A and B provided ratings concerning the prospective success of 100 proposed TV programs. As a scale, the journalists used percent scores that indicated the portion of viewers watching a show. The scale had the six categories $\leq$ 10%; 11 - 20%; 21 - 30%; 31 - 40%; 41 - 50%; and > 50%. Table 2.10 displays the observed frequency distribution.

Table 2.10: **Joint Frequency Distribution of Two TV Journalists' Evaluations of 100 Proposed TV Programs**

		Rater B						
		$\leq$ 10%	11 - 20%	21 - 30%	31 - 40%	41 - 50%	> 50%	Sums
R	$\leq$ 10%	5	8	1	2	4	2	22
a t	11 - 20%	3	5	3	5	5	0	21
e r	21 - 30%	1	2	6	11	2	1	23
A	31 - 40%	0	1	5	4	3	3	16
	41 - 50%	0	0	1	2	5	2	10
	> 50%	0	0	1	2	1	4	8
	Sums	9	16	17	26	20	12	100

To analyze the data in Table 2.10 we first estimate Cohen's κ. We obtain $\kappa = 0.151$, $se_\kappa = 0.054$, $z = 2.796$, and $p = 0.003$. We thus conclude that rater agreement is greater by 15.1% than expected based on chance. This difference may be small, but it is significant. To obtain more detailed information about the structure of the data in this table, we estimate the three hierarchically related log-linear models:

(1)   the main effect base model

$$\log m = \lambda_0 + \lambda_i^A + \lambda_j^B + e,$$

(2)   the equal weight agreement model without linear-by-linear interaction

$$\log m = \lambda_0 + \lambda_i^A + \lambda_j^B + \delta + e,$$

and

(3)   the equal weight agreement model with linear-by-linear interaction

$$\log m = \lambda_0 + \lambda_i^A + \lambda_j^B + \beta u_i u_j + \delta + e.$$

Table 2.11 summarizes the results from these three models. [Note that these models were estimated using SPSS, because Lem (Vermunt, 1997) indicated problems with parameter identification.]

Table 2.11:   Goodness-of-Fit Results for Three Log-Linear Models of Two Journalists' Judgements of 100 TV Programs in Table 2.10

Model	LR-X^2	df	p	ΔX^2 to Model 1; Δdf; p	ΔX^2 to Model 2; Δdf; p
(1)	54.53	25	< 0.01	-	
(2)	44.03	24	0.01	10.50; 1; < 0.01	-
(3)	28.72	23	0.19	25.81; 2; < 0.01	15.31; 1; < 0.01

The results for the three models suggest a strong association between the two journalists' judgements (Model 1). In addition, these results suggest that the equal weight agreement model (Model 2) does not allow one to satisfactorily describe the data in Table 2.10. We conclude that, although rater agreement exceeds chance expectations, there is more going on in this table than can be depicted using δ (or κ) alone. Still, Model 2 represents to a significant improvement over the main effect base model. However, only Model 3 describes the data well.

It is important to realize that the model with linear-by-linear interaction does not introduce an additional substantive hypothesis. Instead, this model uses the information carried by the scale characteristics of the rating variable. Researchers who do not take into account the ordinal nature of rating categories may be tempted to introduce additional substantive hypotheses. The result may be a well fitting model. However, there is the danger of producing models that are unnecessarily complex or, even worse, invalid because substantive information is used to explain what could have been explained from scale characteristics.[5]

The importance of taking scale characteristics into account when specifying a log-linear model in general and for rater agreement in particular can, in the present example, be shown by the model parameters. The parameter for the $\beta u_i u_j$ term is significant. We calculate $\beta = 0.22$, $se_\beta = 0.06$, $z = 3.46$, and $p = 0.0003$. Thus, the linear-by-linear interaction does make a significant contribution to explaining the data in Table 2.10. In contrast, we calculate for $\delta = 0.34$, $se_\delta = 0.25$, $z = 1.35$, and $p = 0.0884$. Therefore, we conclude that the equal weight agreement parameter δ is not significant.

Thus far, we have shown that (a) the two journalists agree to a greater degree than could be expected as chance agreement, (b) taking into consideration the scale level leads to a significant improvement of the log-linear model, and (c) the equal weight agreement hypothesis is only marginally supported, if at all.

Therefore, we ask whether a differential weight agreement model allows one to explain the data better than the equal weight agreement model. We select a new set of weights based on the following consideration. Misjudgements at the scale ends carry the most severe consequences. Misjudgement of lack of spectator interest can result in a loss of large amounts of revenue if a program is not produced that could have been a major success. This applies accordingly for misjudgements of spectator interest. If a program is expected to draw spectator interest but fails, costs can be enormous. Thus, we decided to give larger weights to the extreme ends of the scale and smaller weights to the middle points of the

---

[5] Inversely, of course, there is the danger of producing overly simplistic models when there is not enough power to reject a model that fails to do justice to subtleties present in the data.

rating scale. More specifically, we substituted the weights 1 1 1 1 1 1 in the main diagonal with the weights 3 2 1 1 2 3.

Using these weights in a *differential weight agreement model with linear-by-linear interaction* results in a good description of the data. We calculate LR-$X^2 = 28.19, df = 23, p = 0.209$. These values indicate that there now are no more significant model-data discrepancies. The parameter for the differential weight vector now is $\delta = 0.209$ with $se_\delta = 0.138, z = 1.52$, and $p = 0.0643$. These values indicate that the differential weight hypothesis still fails to make a significant contribution to the explanation of the frequency distribution in Table 2.10. The linear-by-linear interaction parameter is still significant. We obtain $\beta u_i u_j = 0.209$, $se_{\beta u_i u_j} = 0.068$, $z = 3.07$, and $p = 0.001$.

We conclude from these results that the journalists did not assign the proposed differential weights to the ordinal level categories of their evaluations. This result illustrates the benefits that can result from using the more complex log-linear models as compared to simpler and more straightforward measures such as κ or W. From κ we knew that there is agreement beyond chance. However, κ did not give any indication concerning the weights of the six agreement cells. In later sections, we introduce models that involve hypotheses concerning the off-diagonal cells of an $I \times I$ cross-classification. In the following section, we introduce a natural extension of the above model. We introduce the *differential weight agreement model with linear-by-linear interaction with covariates*.

2.3.5 Differential Weight Agreement Model with Linear-by-Linear Interaction plus Covariates

The model that we illustrate in this section is the most complex used thus far. It involves all terms introduced in the general model in Section 2.2. Specifically, we now estimate the complete model

$$\log m = \lambda_0 + \lambda_i^A + \lambda_j^B + \delta + \beta u_i u_j + \lambda^C + e,$$

without setting any of the parameters to zero.

We illustrate this model using a data set presented by Agresti (1992). Two pathologists rated 118 slides that showed samples of carcinoma of the uterine cervix on a four-point ordinal scale with 1 = negative and 4 = invasive carcinoma. The cross-classification of the two raters appears in Table 2.12.

Table 2.12:   **Pathologists' A and B Diagnoses of Severity of Carcinoma**

Pathologist A	Pathologist B			
	1	2	3	4
1	22	2	2	0
2	5	7	14	0
3	0	2	36	0
4	0	1	17	10

In the analysis of the frequency distribution in this table we consider the following variables:

(1)   Pathologist A,
(2)   Pathologist B,
(3)   The differential weight variable δ. In this example, we select the values for δ such that agreement in diagnoses at the extremes of the scale carries more weight than agreement in diagnoses in the middle of the scale. The reason for this determination of weights is that misdiagnoses at the extremes of the scale are probably the most deleterious for patients. Specifically, we specify the weights as 4 for Cells 11 and 44 and 1 for Cells 22 and 33. It should be emphasized that the selection of weights that differ from unity must be carefully justified. Arbitrary selection or selection that optimizes results in one way or the other must be avoided.
(4)   The number of months after diagnosis when the slides were taken. This number is a cell-specific average. (Please note that this variable is artificial. It did not appear in Agresti's analyses.) The averages are row-wise: 1.4, 2.0, 2.2, 0.0, 2.1, 2.2, 2.0, 0.0, 0.0, 2.2, 2.5, 0.0, 0.0, 2.2, 2.3, 1.7.

The complete model for the *differential weight agreement model with linear-by-linear interaction and one covariate* is

$$
\begin{bmatrix}
\log m_{11} \\
\log m_{12} \\
\log m_{13} \\
\log m_{14} \\
\log m_{21} \\
\log m_{22} \\
\log m_{23} \\
\log m_{24} \\
\log m_{31} \\
\log m_{32} \\
\log m_{33} \\
\log m_{34} \\
\log m_{41} \\
\log m_{42} \\
\log m_{43} \\
\log m_{44}
\end{bmatrix}
=
\begin{bmatrix}
1 & 1 & 0 & 0 & 1 & 0 & 0 & 4 & 1 & 1.4 \\
1 & 1 & 0 & 0 & 0 & 1 & 0 & 0 & 2 & 2.0 \\
1 & 1 & 0 & 0 & 0 & 0 & 1 & 0 & 3 & 2.2 \\
1 & 1 & 0 & 0 & -1 & -1 & -1 & 0 & 4 & 0 \\
1 & 0 & 1 & 0 & 1 & 0 & 0 & 0 & 2 & 2.1 \\
1 & 0 & 1 & 0 & 0 & 1 & 0 & 1 & 4 & 2.2 \\
1 & 0 & 1 & 0 & 0 & 0 & 1 & 0 & 6 & 2.0 \\
1 & 0 & 1 & 0 & -1 & -1 & -1 & 0 & 8 & 0 \\
1 & 0 & 0 & 1 & 1 & 0 & 0 & 0 & 3 & 0 \\
1 & 0 & 0 & 1 & 0 & 1 & 0 & 0 & 6 & 2.2 \\
1 & 0 & 0 & 1 & 0 & 0 & 1 & 1 & 9 & 2.5 \\
1 & 0 & 0 & 1 & -1 & -1 & -1 & 0 & 12 & 0 \\
1 & -1 & -1 & -1 & 1 & 0 & 0 & 0 & 4 & 0 \\
1 & -1 & -1 & -1 & 0 & 1 & 0 & 0 & 8 & 2.2 \\
1 & -1 & -1 & -1 & 0 & 0 & 1 & 0 & 12 & 2.3 \\
1 & -1 & -1 & -1 & -1 & -1 & -1 & 4 & 16 & 1.7
\end{bmatrix}
\begin{bmatrix}
\lambda_0 \\
\lambda_1^A \\
\lambda_2^A \\
\lambda_3^A \\
\lambda_1^B \\
\lambda_2^B \\
\lambda_3^B \\
\delta \\
\beta u_i u_j \\
\lambda^C
\end{bmatrix}
+
\begin{bmatrix}
e_{11} \\
e_{12} \\
e_{13} \\
e_{14} \\
e_{21} \\
e_{22} \\
e_{23} \\
e_{24} \\
e_{31} \\
e_{32} \\
e_{33} \\
e_{34} \\
e_{41} \\
e_{42} \\
e_{43} \\
e_{44}
\end{bmatrix}.
$$

We now analyze the pathology agreement data using the four models

(1) The main effect base model $\log m = \lambda_0 + \lambda_i^A + \lambda_j^B + e$. As before, this model does not test any particular hypothesis concerning agreement. However, we use this model as a reference for model comparisons. To be retained, the more specific models must be both tenable by themselves and better than the base model.

(2) The differential weight agreement model, $\log m = \lambda_0 + \lambda_i^A + \lambda_j^B + \delta + e$. This model tests a specific agreement hypothesis (see Section 2.3.1). It is most useful when the rating categories are at the nominal scale level.

(3) The differential weight agreement model with linear-by-linear interaction, $\log m = \lambda_0 + \lambda_i^A + \lambda_j^B + \delta + \beta u_i u_j + e$. This model allows one to consider the ordinal nature of the rating categories.

In the present example, we use the ranks (natural numbers) as scores.

(4)   The differential weight agreement model with linear-by-linear interaction and a covariate,

$$\log m = \lambda_0 + \lambda_i^A + \lambda_j^B + \delta + \beta u_i u_j + \lambda^C + e.$$

This is the complete model. It considers the Covariate *Time at Which the Slide Was Taken* above and beyond the terms considered by the other models.

These four models are hierarchically related to each other. Each higher-numbered model is hierarchically higher than each lower-numbered model. It is clear that a number of additional models could have been considered. Specifically, there are two more models that consider only one of the β, δ, and λ^C terms, and there are three models that include pairs of the β, δ, and λ^C terms. Researchers are encouraged to consider all possible and meaningful models. Table 2.13 displays an overview of the results from the four models considered here.

Table 2.13:   Goodness-of-Fit of Four Models of Two Pathologists' Evaluations (data in Table 2.12)

Model	$LR\text{-}X^2$	df	p	ΔX^2 to Model 1; $\Delta df; p$	ΔX^2 to Model 2; $\Delta df; p$	ΔX^2 to Model 3; $\Delta df; p$
(1)	117.96	9	< 0.01			
(2)	15.14	8	0.057	102.82; 1; < 0.01		
(3)	3.86	7	0.796	114.10; 2; < 0.01	11.28; 1; < 0.01	
(4)	1.00	6	0.986	116.96; 3; < 0.01	14.14; 2; < 0.01	2.86; 1; 0.09

The goodness-of-fit results displayed in Table 2.13 present an interesting pattern. Clearly, the main effect base Model 1 fails to describe the data well. Taking into account only the vector for the differential weight agreement hypothesis leads to a dramatic and significant improvement. The differential weight agreement Model 2 describes the data well and is thus tenable. In principle, researchers could stop at this point because they have identified an interpretable model for which model-data discrepancies are no more than random. However, this model treats the variables as if they were at the nominal scale level. Therefore, we added the linear-by-linear interaction term in Model 3. This model again represents a significant improvement over the differential weight agreement model. The overall LR-X^2 is very small. Model 3 is less parsimonious than Model 2. However, because of the significant improvement, we retain Model 3. Considering the very low LR-X^2 of Model 3, fitting Model 4 is a mere exercise. A LR-X^2 of 3.86 can be significantly reduced only if the X^2-value goes down to practically zero [p(X^2 = 3.86; df = 1) = 0.04945]. Accordingly, Model 4 is only non-significantly better than Model 3. It would be tenable by itself. However, because it is less parsimonious than Model 3 and not significantly better, we retain Model 3.

The δ and β parameters in Model 3 are both significant. Specifically, we calculate δ = 0.45, se_δ = 0.21, z = 2.10, and p_δ = 0.0357; β = 1.18, se_β = 0.44, z = 2.66, and p_β = 0.0078. We thus conclude that the differential weight hypothesis is confirmed for the particular weights used in this analysis. In addition, the linear-by-linear interaction makes a significant contribution to the explanation of these data. The artificial covariate is not needed to describe the data.

2.4   Extensions

This section presents extensions that go beyond the typical application of models of rater agreement. Specifically, extensions are discussed that involve (1) more than two raters and (2) rater-specific trends.

2.4.1   Modeling Agreement among More than Two Raters

In many studies, researchers employ three or more raters with the goal of estimating the variability of ratings from a random sample of raters. The present section is concerned with modeling agreement between small numbers of raters. Each of these raters examines many objects. In an analogous fashion, models can be devised for situations in which many raters examine small numbers of objects, or many raters examine many objects. We consider two types of models for the sample case of three raters. The first type simultaneously estimates rater agreement for all three pairs of raters. The second type of model considers the agreement among all three raters.

2.4.1.1 Estimation of Rater-Pair-Specific Parameters

Consider the three raters, A, B, and C. Each of these raters makes n decisions concerning a set of n objects. Each decision is scored on a I-point scale. The cross-classification of all three raters' decisions has I_A x I_B x I_C cells where the subscripts index the raters. For the examples in this text, we only consider cases where the raters use the same categories, that is, $I_A = I_B = I_C$. The cross-classification I_A x I_B describes the joint use of rating categories of Raters A and B. The cross-classification I_A x I_C describes the joint use of rating categories of Raters A and C, and I_B x I_C describes the joint use of categories of Raters B and C.

To simultaneously assess the agreement between the $\binom{n_r}{2}$ pairs of raters, where n_r is the number of raters, we use, for $n_r = 3$, the extended Tanner and Young (1985, p. 176) model

$$\log m = \lambda_0 + \lambda_i^A + \lambda_j^B + \lambda_k^C + \delta^{AB} + \delta^{AC} + \delta^{BC} + e,$$

with $i, j, k = 1, ..., I$ and $I = I_A = I_B = I_C$. When there are more than three raters, the model can be extended accordingly.

Data example. To illustrate this model, we use data from the depression diagnoses study again (cf. Section 2.3.3.2). We use three different psychiatrists than in Table 1.2 and a different patient pool. Each rater processed the same 163 patient files. For the following analyses we use equal weights. That is, $\delta^{AB} = \delta^{AC} = \delta^{BC}$ and, specifically, $\delta_{1,1,.} = \delta_{2,2,.} = ... = \delta_{I,I,.}$, $\delta_{1,.,1} = \delta_{2,.,2} = ... = \delta_{I,.,I}$, and $\delta_{.,1,1} = \delta_{.,2,2} = ... = \delta_{.,I,I}$. The 3 x 3 x 3 cross-classification of the three raters' responses appears in Table 2.14. The three subtables in Table 2.14 display the cross-classifications of Rater B with Rater C for the ratings given by Rater A. For example, the cross-classification of the ratings of Raters B and C appears in the first subtable, which contains all patients for which Rater A assigned a 1. The tables suggest that Rater A used rating category 1 (no depression) 40 times. He/she used Category 2 (non-clinical depression) 10 times, and Category 3 (clinical depression) 113 times.

Table 2.14: Three Psychiatrists' Re-Diagnoses of Psychiatric Patients

Rater A = 1		Rater C			
		1	2	3	Total
Rater B	1	4	3	6	13
	2	2	1	3	6
	3	2	2	17	21
	Total	8	6	26	40

Rater A = 2		Rater C			
		1	2	3	Total
Rater B	1	0	1	2	3
	2	1	1	1	3
	3	0	0	4	4
	Total	1	2	7	10

Rater A = 3		Rater C			
		1	2	3	Total
Rater B	1	0	1	3	4
	2	0	1	8	9
	3	0	4	96	100
	Total	0	6	107	113

We now analyze the data in this table using two models:

(1)   The base main effect-only model. This is the model

$$\log m = \lambda_0 + \lambda_i^A + \lambda_j^B + \lambda_k^C + e.$$

As before, we need this model for a reference.

(2)   The model of simultaneous agreement between pairs of raters given above:

$$\log m = \lambda_0 + \lambda_i^A + \lambda_j^B + \lambda_k^C + \delta^{AB} + \delta^{AC} + \delta^{BC} + e.$$

The design matrix for the second model is

$$X = \begin{bmatrix}
1 & 1 & 0 & 1 & 0 & 1 & 0 & 1 & 1 & 1 \\
1 & 1 & 0 & 1 & 0 & 0 & 1 & 1 & 0 & 0 \\
1 & 1 & 0 & 1 & 0 & -1 & -1 & 1 & 0 & 0 \\
1 & 1 & 0 & 0 & 1 & 1 & 0 & 0 & 1 & 0 \\
1 & 1 & 0 & 0 & 1 & 0 & 1 & 0 & 0 & 1 \\
1 & 1 & 0 & 0 & 1 & -1 & -1 & 0 & 0 & 0 \\
1 & 1 & 0 & -1 & -1 & 1 & 0 & 0 & 1 & 0 \\
1 & 1 & 0 & -1 & -1 & 0 & 1 & 0 & 0 & 0 \\
1 & 1 & 0 & -1 & -1 & -1 & -1 & 0 & 0 & 1 \\
1 & 0 & 1 & 1 & 0 & 1 & 0 & 0 & 0 & 1 \\
1 & 0 & 1 & 1 & 0 & 0 & 1 & 0 & 1 & 0 \\
1 & 0 & 1 & 1 & 0 & -1 & -1 & 0 & 0 & 0 \\
1 & 0 & 1 & 0 & 1 & 1 & 0 & 1 & 0 & 0 \\
1 & 0 & 1 & 0 & 1 & 0 & 1 & 1 & 1 & 1 \\
1 & 0 & 1 & 0 & 1 & -1 & -1 & 1 & 0 & 0 \\
1 & 0 & 1 & -1 & -1 & 1 & 0 & 0 & 0 & 0 \\
1 & 0 & 1 & -1 & -1 & 0 & 1 & 0 & 1 & 0 \\
1 & 0 & 1 & -1 & -1 & -1 & -1 & 0 & 0 & 1 \\
1 & -1 & -1 & 1 & 0 & 1 & 0 & 0 & 0 & 1 \\
1 & -1 & -1 & 1 & 0 & 0 & 1 & 0 & 0 & 0 \\
1 & -1 & -1 & 1 & 0 & -1 & -1 & 0 & 1 & 0 \\
1 & -1 & -1 & 0 & 1 & 1 & 0 & 0 & 0 & 0 \\
1 & -1 & -1 & 0 & 1 & 0 & 1 & 0 & 0 & 1 \\
1 & -1 & -1 & 0 & 1 & -1 & -1 & 0 & 1 & 0 \\
1 & -1 & -1 & -1 & -1 & 1 & 0 & 1 & 0 & 0 \\
1 & -1 & -1 & -1 & -1 & 0 & 1 & 1 & 0 & 0 \\
1 & -1 & -1 & -1 & -1 & -1 & -1 & 1 & 1 & 1
\end{bmatrix}$$

The first column in this design matrix is the constant, for the intercept. The second and third columns represent the two main effect parameters for Rater A. The fourth and fifth columns represent the main effects for Rater B. The sixth and seventh columns represent the main effects for Rater C. The last three columns represent the equal weight agreement hypotheses for the three pairs of raters, Raters A and B, Raters A and C, and Raters B and C, respectively.

For the base model, we calculate a LR-$X^2 = 75.10$ ($df = 20; p < 0.01$). Based on this result, this model is not tenable.[6] The base model contains all vectors in the design matrix except the last three. In contrast, the model of simultaneous agreement between pairs of raters for which we use the entire design matrix, yields a very good fit with LR-$X^2 = 17.97$, $df = 17$, and $p = 0.391$. The estimates for the parameters for the three pairwise agreement assessments are $\delta^{AB} = 0.99$ ($se = 0.23; p < 0.01$), $\delta^{AC} = 1.10$ ($se = 0.31; p < 0.01$), and $\delta^{BC} = 0.71$ ($se = 0.28; p = 0.016$), respectively. However, while the overall fit is good, and the equal weight agreement hypothesis for each rater pair makes a significant contribution to the explanation of the frequency distribution in Table 2.14, there may be room for improvement. Specifically, one may ask whether considering the agreement among all three raters leads to an improved model fit. In the next section, we show how to model the agreement among all three raters.

2.4.1.2   Agreement among Three Raters

In order to also consider the information carried by the agreement among all three raters, we add the term δ^{ABC} to the above model. This term represents those cells where all three raters agree, specifically, Cells 111, 222, and 333. The corresponding vector is $x' = [1, 0, 0, 0, 0, 0, 0, 0, 0, 0, 0, 0, 0, 1, 0, 0, 0, 0, 0, 0, 0, 0, 0, 0, 0, 0, 1]$. The model that includes this term improves the model from Section 2.4.1.1 only modestly. We calculate LR-$X^2 = 17.55$ ($df = 16; p = 0.35$). This improvement is nonsignificant ($\Delta X^2 = 0.42; \Delta df = 1; p = 0.517$). In addition, none of the parameters that represent rater agreement is significant any more.

One interpretation of this last result is that the vector that represents the agreement among all three raters and the vectors that represent pairwise

---

[6] Notice that some of the estimated expected cell frequencies for this base model are that small that there would be reason to be very cautious even if the base model were tenable.

agreement exhaust the same information. To give credence to this interpretation, we also estimated a model that includes only the vector for the agreement among all three raters. The fit of this model is very good. One obtains LR-X^2 = 20.89 (df = 19; p = 0.3427). The difference to the more complete model that also considers the pairwise, equal-weight agreement patterns is not significant (ΔX^2 = 3.34; Δdf = 3; p = 0.3421). Of the three models that evaluate the agreement among three raters the one that only considers the agreement between all three raters is the most parsimonious. We therefore retain this model, and conclude that knowledge of the agreement of all three raters is sufficient to explain the variability in the data that is observed beyond what the main effects allow one to explain. Knowledge of agreement in the three pairs of raters does not provide additional explanatory power.

Further extensions. The three-rater agreement model that we retained has 19 degrees of freedom. Thus, there is plenty of room for additional specifications. Examples of such specifications include the association measurement models discussed above, models that group raters if there exist specific dependency patterns, models with differential agreement weights, or models with covariates. In addition, models can be considered with rater-specific trends. Examples of such trend models are introduced in the next section.

2.4.2 Rater-Specific Trends

Students are often suspected of gravitating toward those examiners that are believed to exhibit such trends as leniency. In rater agreement studies, examiners with leniency tendencies tend not to agree with examiners without such trend. However, knowledge of such a trend would explain the association between raters' judgements. This section presents a model for raters who are hypothesized to differ systematically. The model decomposes the variability in a cross-classification of two raters' responses in three parts (Goodman, 1984; Meiser, von Eye, & Spiel, 1997). The first part includes intercept and main effects. This is the base model. The second part includes the agreement as reflected in the main diagonal. The third part models the trend that one rater may be more lenient (or strict). This trend manifests in an increased number of responses above (below) the main diagonal of the cross-classification. Thus, the model has the same form as the covariate model given in Section 2.3.3.2. The covariate specifies the trend. The model to be fit is

$$\log\ m\ =\ \lambda_0\ +\ \lambda_i^A\ +\ \lambda_j^B\ +\ \delta\ +\ \lambda^C\ +\ e.$$

To illustrate this model, we use the data from Section 2.3.3.2, and ask whether Psychiatrist A (rows) has a tendency to view patients as less paranoid than Psychiatrist B (columns). If this trend exists, the cell frequencies above the diagonal in the 3 x 3 cross-classification are larger than their counterparts below the diagonal. The cross-classification of the two psychiatrists' diagnoses is given in Table 2.15.

We analyze the data in Table 2.15 using (1) the base model of only main effects and (2) the equal weight agreement model in which we include the additional hypothesis that Psychiatrist A has a trend toward lower paranoia ratings. The design matrix for this model is

$$X = \begin{bmatrix} 1 & 1 & 0 & 1 & 0 & 1 & 0 \\ 1 & 1 & 0 & 0 & 1 & 0 & 1 \\ 1 & 1 & 0 & -1 & -1 & 0 & 1 \\ 1 & 0 & 1 & 1 & 0 & 0 & -1 \\ 1 & 0 & 1 & 0 & 1 & 1 & 0 \\ 1 & 0 & 1 & -1 & -1 & 0 & 1 \\ 1 & -1 & -1 & 1 & 0 & 0 & -1 \\ 1 & -1 & -1 & 0 & 1 & 0 & -1 \\ 1 & -1 & -1 & -1 & -1 & 1 & 0 \end{bmatrix}$$

The last vector in this design matrix reflects the hypothesis that the frequencies above the diagonal are greater than the frequencies below the diagonal. More specifically, the cells above the diagonal are assigned a 1, and the cells below the diagonal are assigned a -1. The cells above the diagonal have the indices 12, 13, and 23. The cells below the diagonal have the indices 21, 31, and 32. The diagonal cells are not part of this hypothesis. The data for this model appear in Table 2.15.

Cohen's κ for this data set is $\hat{\kappa} = 0.11$, indicating that rater agreement exceeds chance agreement by 11%. The standard error for $\hat{\kappa}$ is $s\hat{e}_\kappa = 0.073, z = 1.51$, and $p = 0.066$. This result suggests that the two raters fail to agree in their paranoia ratings better than chance. We now ask whether an equal weight agreement model with trend hypothesis allows one to describe these data in more detail.

Table 2.15:   Cross-Classification of Two Psychiatrists' Paranoia Ratings

		Psychiatrist B: Severity of Paranoia		
		1	2	3	Sums
Psychiatrist A: Severity of Paranoia	1	17	27	3	47
	2	16	45	14	75
	3	1	3	3	7
	Sums	34	75	20	$N = 129$

The results for the main effect base model indicate that this model already describes the data well (LR-X^2 = 9.10; df = 4; p = 0.059). However, there may be room for improvement. The equal weight agreement model with the trend hypothesis yields LR-X^2 = 3.46 (df = 2; p = 0.18). None of the residuals is larger than z = 2. The parameter for the main diagonal is estimated as δ = 0.37 (se_δ = 0.20; z = 1.80; p = 0.08). The parameter for the trend is estimated as λ^t = 0.82 (se_t = 0.48; z = 1.70; p = 0.09). Neither parameter suggests that significant portions of variability have been captured. In addition, the ΔX^2 = 5.64 (df = 2; p = 0.06) suggests that the equal weight agreement model with the trend hypothesis is not significantly better than the main effect base model. Therefore, we retain the more parsimonious model of independence. The hypotheses of equal weight agreement and a trend towards lower paranoia scores given by Psychiatrist A are left unconfirmed.

More models are conceivable. For instance, one can devise models based on the assumption that one of the raters uses rank $r + 1$ when the other rater uses rank r (for $r < I$). In addition, one can consider covariates or the ordinal nature of the rating categories. These and other considerations can be taken into account simultaneously, if there are enough degrees of freedom.

2.4.3 Generalized Coefficients κ

An interesting option to come to closure concerning results created using log-linear models and coefficients of agreement involves estimating generalized κ coefficients. In Section 1.1, we defined κ as a measure that describes rater agreement beyond chance, $\kappa = (\theta_1 - \theta_2)/(1 - \theta_2)$. The reference values for θ_2 were estimated using such base models as the main effect log-linear model of rater (or object) independence. Now, the null model used for Brennan and Prediger's (1991) coefficient and the models presented in this chapter can be viewed as alternative base models. In fact, each of the models discussed in this chapter represents a particular base model. If this model describes the data well, any κ will be rather small. If the model fails to describe the data well, κ will be large. In either case, a κ coefficient will indicate the degree to which there is agreement above and beyond what was proposed by the base model.

One characteristic of the chance models used for Cohen's κ or Brennan and Prediger's κ_n is that researchers typically do not expect that the base models for the coefficients allow them to explain the data well. The reason for this expectation is that the chance models do not contain a substantive hypothesis about the data that could be used to explain agreement. In contrast, the models used in this chapter do contain substantive hypotheses. Therefore, the interpretation of generalized κ coefficients differs in its meaning from the interpretation of the original coefficients. Interpretation of generalized coefficients focuses on the portions of agreement and disagreement that are left unexplained when a particular substantive hypothesis is tested using a particular model which includes specific propositions about the agreement structure. In contrast, the interpretation of coefficients that arc calculated on models with no substantive hypothesis, such as the main effect or the null models, allows one only to test the null hypothesis that agreement is no better than chance.

Data examples. To illustrate the use of generalized κ coefficients, we re-analyze data that were discussed by Lawal (2003; p. 488/9). A sample of 69 multiple sclerosis patients in New Orleans were re-diagnosed by a neurologist from Winnipeg. The diagnoses from the neurologists in New Orleans and Winnipeg were then compared and assessed for agreement. A four point Likert scale was used for diagnosis with 1 indicating certain multiple sclerosis, 2 indicating probable multiple sclerosis, 3 indicating possible multiple sclerosis, and 4 indicating doubtful, unlikely, or definitely not multiple sclerosis. Table 2.16 presents the cross-classification of these diagnoses.

Table 2.16: **Comparative Diagnoses for Multiple Sclerosis Patients (expected cell frequencies, estimated for differential weight agreement model, in *italics*)**

New Orleans neurologist	Winnipeg neurologist				
	1	2	3	4	Totals
1	5	3	0	0	8
	5.11	*1.81*	*0.64*	*0.45*	
2	3	11	4	0	18
	1.89	*11.73*	*2.58*	*1.80*	
3	2	13	3	4	22
	2.74	*10.59*	*6.05*	*2.62*	
4	1	2	4	14	21
	1.26	*4.87*	*1.73*	*13.14*	
Totals	11	29	11	18	69

Cohen's κ for the cross-classification in Table 2.16 is 0.297 (se = 0.079; $p < 0.01$). This value suggests that the two neurologists agree to almost 30% better than chance, a significant value. Raw agreement is 47.83%, a rather small value. To illustrate the use of generalized κ coefficients, we now ask whether a differential agreement model allows one to describe the data in Table 2.16 well. We assume that misdiagnoses at the extremes of the scales are most problematic and select the following weights: 5 for Cells 1 1 and 4 4, and 1 for Cells 2 2 and 3 3. Table 2.17 presents the results for the base model of rater independence and the differential weight agreement model.

Table 2.17: **Results for the Base Model and the Differential Weight Agreement Model for the Data in Table 2.16**

Model	X^2	$df; p$	ΔX^2	$\Delta df; p$
base model	46.264	9; < .01		
diff. weights	14.430	8; .051	31.834	1; < .01

The results in Table 2.17 show that the base model fails to describe the diagnostic data well. In contrast, the differential weight agreement model (a) presents a significant improvement over the base model and (b) is tenable by itself. However, although this model can be retained, there seems to be variability that is left unexplained. We now calculate the generalized κ to determine if the agreement cells carry information that the model fails to capture. Using the expected cell frequencies from Table 2.16, we estimate the generalized kappa as

$$\hat{\kappa} = \frac{(5+11+3+14)/69 \ - \ (5.11+11.73+6.05+13.14)/69}{1 \ - \ (5.11+11.73+6.05+13.14)/69}$$

$$= \frac{0.478 \ - \ 0.522}{1 \ - \ 0.522} \ = \ -0.092.$$

This generalized κ score shows an interesting result. The differential weight agreement model *over*estimated the degree to which the two neurologists propose the same diagnoses by almost 10%. We thus can conclude that while the differential weight agreement model does allow one to state that the extreme diagnostic categories carry much heavier weights than the categories about the midpoint of the scale, this model met with agreement frequencies that were smaller than proposed.

Note. In the following paragraphs, we give a second example. This example illustrates that the generalized coefficient κ cannot be meaningfully applied to the equal weight agreement model. More specifically, the equal weight agreement model comes with weights for the cells in the main diagonal of a cross-classification that have the effect that the sum of the estimated expected frequencies in the agreement cells are always equal to the sum of the observed frequencies in the agreement cells. As a consequence, the numerator of generalized κ will always be zero, when the equal weight agreement model is used. Consider the following illustration.

An example of a situation in which κ and the log-linear analyses suggested discrepant conclusions was presented by von Eye and Schuster (2000; see Table 1.2, above). In the study on the reliability of psychiatric diagnoses, two psychiatrists re-evaluated the files of $N = 129$ inpatients that had previously been diagnosed as clinically depressed. The psychiatrists evaluated the severity of the patients' depression. The data in Table 2.18 describe the ratings that the two raters provided. The rating categories were 1 = not depressed, 2 = mildly depressed, and 3 = clinically depressed. In the following analysis we ask whether (1) the two raters agree beyond chance, and (2) whether the agreement is statistically significantly greater than could be expected from chance.

Table 2.18:   **Two Psychiatrists' Perception of Severity of Depression (expected cell frequencies, estimated based on equal weight agreement model, in *italics*)**

		Psychiatrist 2: Severity of Depression			Row Sums
		1	2	3	
Psychiatrist 1: Severity of Depression	1	11 *9.443*	2 *4.635*	19 *17.921*	32
	2	1 *0.363*	3 *3.557*	3 *3.080*	7
	3	0 *2.193*	8 *4.807*	82 *82.990*	90
Column Sums		12	13	104	$N = 129$

For the main effect model of data in Table 2.18 we calculate a LR-X^2 = 39.03 ($df = 4$; $p < 0.01$) and $\hat{\kappa}$ = 0.375 ($\hat{se}_\kappa$ = 0.079; $z = 5.943$; $p < 0.01$). We thus conclude that (1) the assumption of independence between these two raters' perceptions can be rejected; (2) the raters' agreement is 37.5% greater than was expected based on chance; and (3) the agreement between the two raters is significantly better than chance.

In contrast, when applying the equal weight agreement model, we obtain an LR-X^2 = 9.22; $df = 3$; and $p = 0.0265$. We thus reject this model with reference to the usual $\alpha = 0.05$, and cannot interpret the δ parameter. The reason for this result is that the model, overall, does not describe the data well. While none of the individual residuals is exorbitantly large, there are several that are close to being significant, in particular among the off-diagonal cells. Thus, the equal weight agreement model must be rejected.

Calculating a generalized κ coefficient based on the expected frequencies that resulted for the equal weight agreement model (see Table 2.3), we obtain the interesting estimate

$$\hat{\kappa} = \frac{(11+3+82)/129 - (9.443+3.557+82.990)/129}{1 - (9.443+3.557+82.990)/129} = 0.000.$$

This value of zero is not an empirical result. It does not describe data characteristics. It is zero solely because the sum of the estimated expected cell frequencies in the agreement cells, and the sum of the observed frequencies in these cells are always the same in the equal weight agreement model.

Thus, we can only conclude from the estimate of κ from the rater-independence base model that (1) the two psychiatrists agree beyond chance, and (2) that the equal weight hypothesis does not allow us to explain the frequency distribution in Table 2.3. The generalized κ does not provide us with additional information, in this case.

2.5 Exercises

2-1. Using the table created to answer exercise question 1-5, run the following four log-linear models: (1) main-effect base model, (2) equal weight agreement model, (3) differential weight agreement model, and (4) equal weight agreement model with a covariate for linear-by-linear association. For the differential weight log-linear model, use weights 1, 2, 3 for the diagonal cells and zeros for the off-diagonal cells. Which is the best and most parsimonious agreement model of all four? What does it say about the data?

2-2. Using the data in Table 1.6, run the log-linear models of (1) rater independence (i.e., main-effect base model), (2) rater-pair-specific agreement, and (3) agreement among all three raters in a hierarchical way (see Section 2.4). Compare the model fits and interpret results.

2-3. The following observed frequencies are from a study by Furman, Simon, Shaffer, and Bouchey (2002), in which adolescents' relationships with parents, friends, and romantic partners were classified into three categories: Secure, Preoccupied, and Dismissing. Based on Cohen's κ, it appears that the relationship style with parents and friends carries over to the relationship with romantic partners only modestly ($\hat{\kappa}$ = .14 and .36, respectively). Using parents/friends as a stratum variable, test the log-linear models of (1) main-effect base model, and (2) equal weight model including pair-wise associations with the stratum variable. Compare the model fits. Which model explains the data better and why?

	Relationship with Romantic Partners		
	Secure	Preoccupied	Dismissing
Relationship with Parents			
Secure	18	2	4
Preoccupied	1	2	0
Dismissing	23	5	10
Relationship with Friends			
Secure	24	4	3
Preoccupied	3	7	1
Dismissing	15	0	10

2-4.   The data by Jackson and her colleagues (2001) presented in question 1-7 are broken down into two groups: one with family history of alcoholism and the rest without family history of alcoholism. Analyze the data using the following four log-linear models and compare them.

(1)   The main effect base model,

$$\log m = \lambda_0 + \lambda_i^F + \lambda_j^{W1} + \lambda_k^{W2} + e.$$

(2)   The equal weight agreement without the triple-superscripted association term,

$$\log m = \lambda_0 + \lambda_i^F + \lambda_j^{W1} + \lambda_k^{W2} + \lambda_{ij}^{F,W1} + \lambda_{ik}^{F,W2} + \delta^{W1,W2} + e.$$

(3)   The equal weight agreement with the linear by linear association term,

$$\log m = \lambda_0 + \lambda_i^F + \lambda_j^{W1} + \lambda_k^{W2} + \lambda_{ij}^{F,W1} + \lambda_{ik}^{F,W2} + \delta^{W1,W2} + \beta u_j u_k + e.$$

(4)   The model (3) with the λ^C for one continuous covariate. For the continuous covariate, use $X_c' = [.56, .23, .17, .03, .10, .37, .46, .07, .05, .30, .40, .24, .04, .01, .23, .71]$. This vector consists of proportions of transition from W1 to W2 derived from question 1.7.

Freshmen (W1)	Three Years Later (W2)			
	Abstainer (1)	Limited-effect Drinker (2)	Moderate-effect Drinker (3)	Large-effect Drinker (4)
Family history of alcoholism (F)				
1	20	8	3	2
2	6	8	3	2
3	2	13	8	10
4	9	8	27	96
No family history of alcoholism (F)				
1	13	8	6	0
2	0	6	13	1
3	3	13	26	15
4	3	0	26	84

3.   Exploring Rater Agreement

The methods discussed in Chapters 1 and 2 are typically employed in explanatory contexts. Researchers are interested in the degree of rater agreement, in the effects of covariates, in the comparison of groups of objects, or in the comparisons of raters and groups of raters. The resulting statements are general in the sense that they refer to parameters that describe agreement and the structure of agreement in general. For instance, the parameter δ provides information about the entire main diagonal.

However, there exist instances in which researchers are interested in exploring whether the degree of agreement or disagreement varies across the rating categories, or whether agreement exists in some categories but not in others. In addition, researchers may be interested in configurations of rating categories that indicate agreement or disagreement beyond chance.

Configural Frequency Analysis (CFA; Lienert & Krauth, 1975; von Eye, 2002a) is a method for the exploration of cross-classifications. CFA allows one to inspect individual cells and to answer the question whether a cell contains more or fewer cases than expected based on some chance model. The following section provides a brief introduction to CFA. Exploratory applications of CFA to cross-classifications of rater agreement are presented in the subsequent sections.

3.1   Configural Frequency Analysis: A Tutorial

Consider a cross-classification of $I \times I = c$ cells. The observed frequency of Cell i in this table is m_i, where i goes over all cells in the table. The expected frequency that is estimated for Cell i based on some chance model is $\hat{m}_i$. CFA asks for each i, whether m_i differs from $\hat{m}_i$. The null hypothesis for each cell-wise test is H_o: $E[m_i] = \hat{m}_i$, where E indicates the *expectancy*. If $m_i > \hat{m}_i$, Cell i is said to constitute a *CFA type*. If $m_i < \hat{m}_i$, Cell i is said to constitute a *CFA antitype*. If there is no statistically significant difference between m_i and $\hat{m}_i$, Cell i constitutes neither a type nor an antitype.[7]   Types suggests that the frequency in Cell i is significantly greater than expected based on the chance model used to estimate $\hat{m}_i$. Antitypes suggest that the frequency in Cell i is significantly smaller than expected based on the chance model used to estimate $\hat{m}_i$.

CFA chance models reflect assumptions that are contradicted by the existence of types and antitypes. For example, if the chance model proposes independence between the variables that span a cross-classification, types and antitypes suggest that the variables are associated, at least locally, that is, in particular sectors of the cross-classification (Havránek & Lienert, 1984).

In principle, any model that allows one to derive expected probabilities for a cross-classification can serve as a CFA chance model. Constraints result mostly from sampling schemes and from interpretational issues (von Eye & Schuster, 1998a). Four groups of base models have been discussed in the CFA literature (von Eye, 2002, 2004). The first and most frequently employed groups includes hierarchical log-linear models. These are standard log-linear models which take main effects and variable interactions into account. The role of these models in CFA is to estimate the expected cell frequencies according to the specifications made in some base model. Estimation typically uses maximum likelihood methods and the observed marginal frequencies. The second group of base models estimates the expected cell frequencies using population parameters rather than observed marginal frequencies. The third group of base models uses theoretically derived, a priori probabilities for the estimation of the expected cell frequencies. Groups two and three of base models are not

---

[7] A similar approach, with a focus on what is here called a type, was described by DuMouchel (1999) in the context of Bayesian exploration of large contingency tables.

necessarily log-linear. The fourth group estimates the expected cell frequencies based on distributional assumptions. This group of base models is practically never log-linear.

In the present context, however, we focus on log-linear base models of the kind given above. More specifically, we ask whether the agreement between two raters results in types in the main diagonal of an I x I cross-classification, and in antitypes in the off-diagonal cells. More detail follows in the sections below.

There exists a large number of statistical tests that can be used for the comparison of m_i with $\hat{m}_i$. Most popular are the binomial test and Pearson's X^2 test. The binomial test allows one to estimate the tail probability B_i of the observed frequency, m_i, of Cell i, given the probability, p, expected for this cell from some base model and the sample size, N. The tail probability B_i can be calculated as follows. For a CFA chance model, the expected probability for Cell i is estimated as $p_i = \hat{m}_i / N$, where i indexes the cells of the cross-classification, also called *configurations*. Then, the tail probability for the observed frequency, m_i, and more extreme frequencies is

$$B_i(m_i) = \sum_{j=a}^{l} \binom{N}{j} p_i^j q_i^{N-j},$$

where i indexes the cells of the cross-classification, $q = 1 - p$, and

$$a = \begin{cases} 0 & \text{if } m_i < \hat{m}_i \\ m_i & \text{if } m_i \geq \hat{m}_i \end{cases},$$

and

$$l = \begin{cases} m_i & \text{if } a = 0 \\ N & \text{if } a = m_i \end{cases}.$$

The binomial test has a number of characteristics that make it interesting for use in CFA. First, the test is nonparametric. Thus, there is no need to make distributional assumptions, and there is no need to test such assumptions. Second, the test is exact. As can be seen in the formula for B_i, the point probabilities for the observed frequencies and each of the more extreme frequencies are calculated and summed. Thus, there is no need to assume that a test statistic is sufficiently near to some sampling distribution. B_i is the desired tail probability itself.

However, the test can also be conservative. If p is estimated using sample information, one can assume that p is closer to the data than if it were based on population information.

When the expected cell frequency is large enough, that is, when $\hat{m}_i$ ≥ 10, the binomial can be approximated by the normal distribution. One obtains the standard normally distributed test statistic

$$z = \frac{m_i - \hat{m}_i}{\sqrt{\hat{m}_i(1 - p_i)}} .$$

The Pearson X^2 test uses the test statistic

$$X^2 = \frac{(m_i - \hat{m}_i)^2}{\hat{m}_i} ,$$

with $df = 1$. This test is computationally simpler than the exact binomial test. However, it tends to suggest more conservative type-antitype decisions, in particular in the search for antitypes in small samples (von Eye, 2002a).

When, as is routine in exploratory CFA, all c cells of a cross-classification are subjected to significance tests, the nominal significance level α must be protected. There are two reasons why the factual level α can differ from the nominal level α. The first reason is that *tests can be dependent*. If CFA finds significantly more cases than expected in a particular cell, then there must be fewer cases than expected in one or more cells, because the sample size N (or the row marginals or the column marginals under product-multinomial sampling) is given. In extreme cases, the existence of a type predetermines the existence of an antitype, and vice versa. The second reason is known as *capitalizing on chance*. When c tests are performed on the same sample, the probability of committing an error is α for each test. As a consequence, one can expect $c \cdot \alpha$ type-antitype decisions to be incorrect.

For these two reasons, protection of the significance level α is part of all CFA applications. The classical method for α protection is called Bonferroni's method. Let α_i be the α error of the test of the ith cell frequency, for i, ..., c, and let α^* be the probability that at least one of the c tests leads to falsely rejecting the null hypothesis that no type or antitype exists. Then, the Bonferroni method controls the significance level α such that two conditions are fulfilled. First, the sum of all values α_i does not exceed the nominal α. In different words,

$$\sum_{i=1}^{c} \alpha_i \leq \alpha.$$

Second, the Bonferroni method determines the α_i such that they are all equal, or

$$\alpha_i = \alpha^* \quad for\ all\ i = 1, ..., c.$$

In this equation, α^* is called the *adjusted* α, that is, the value for the significance threshold that fulfills both conditions specified by Bonferroni's method. This value is

$$\alpha^* = \alpha/c .$$

In CFA significance testing, the one-sided tail probabilities of the cell-wise significance tests are compared with the adjusted threshold, α^*, rather than the nominal threshold, α. To illustrate the Bonferroni adjustment, consider a 6 x 6 cross-classification. If each cell in this table is subjected to CFA and the nominal significance level is $\alpha = 0.05$, the Bonferroni-adjusted α is $\alpha^* = 0.05/36 = 0.001389$.

The Bonferroni procedure is known to suggest conservative decisions. Therefore, in the present context of 2-dimensional tables, a procedure proposed by Hommel, Lehmacher, and Perli (1985; cf. Hommel, 1988) is often preferred. This method is far more powerful, that is, it is less prohibitive in the search for types and antitypes. This procedure uses adjusted levels α_i^* that are not constant for all cells i. In addition, this procedure exploits the dependence structure of tests in 2-dimensional tables and therefore allows groups of tests to be performed at the same adjusted significance thresholds, most of which are less extreme than Bonferroni's adjusted threshold, and none of which is more extreme than Bonferroni's. The series of adjusted significance thresholds is

$$\alpha_1^* = \alpha_2^* = ... = \alpha_5^* = \frac{\alpha}{c - 4} ,$$

$$\alpha_6^* = \alpha_7^* = \frac{\alpha}{c - 6} ,$$

$$\alpha_8^* = \frac{\alpha}{c - 7} ,$$

$$\alpha_{c-1}^* = \frac{\alpha}{2} ,$$

and

$$\alpha_c^* = \alpha .$$

Obviously, this procedure yields less restrictive adjusted significance thresholds already for the first test, α_i^*. Extensions of this procedure for three-way tables have been proposed by Perli, Hommel, and Lehmacher (1985), alternative procedures have been presented, for instance, by Keselman, Cribbie, and Holland (1999).

In the application to rater agreement data, CFA proceeds in four steps. The first step involves specifying a base model. With a few exceptions, the same base models can be used as for the log-linear analysis of rater agreement data. Exceptions include the models with the parameters δ, that is, the parameters used to model the agreement cells in the main diagonal. In contrast to log-linear modeling, it is not the goal of CFA to describe the data using a model. Instead, CFA identifies those cells that deviate significantly from some base model. If raters agree significantly beyond chance, the agreement cells should emerge as types, and at least some of the disagreement cells should emerge as antitypes.

The second step of CFA of agreement data involves the estimation of expected cell frequencies. In the present context and with the focus on log-linear base models, the same methods can be used as for log-linear modeling.

The third step involves identifying types and antitypes. The first part of this step involves employing the procedures for the protection of the significance threshold α introduced above. The second part of this step involves employing the CFA significance tests (for more tests see von Eye, 2002a). The fourth and last step involves interpreting the emerging types and antitypes. The following sections present sample applications using various base models.

In the context of an exploration of rater agreement, CFA types and antitypes can emerge as follows (von Eye & Mun, 2004):

(1)   *Agreement types* in cells in the main diagonal of an agreement table suggest more frequent agreement in particular rating categories than expected by the base model;

(2)   *Agreement antitypes* in cells in the main diagonal of an agreement table suggest less frequent agreement in particular rating categories than expected by the base model;

(3)   *Disagreement types* in off-diagonal cells of an agreement table suggest more frequent disagreement in particular rating categories than expected by the base model; and

(4)   *Disagreement antitypes* in off-diagonal cells of an agreement table suggest less frequent disagreement in particular rating categories than expected by the base model.

3.2　CFA Base Models for Rater Agreement Data

The general log-linear base model for the analysis of rater agreement given in Section 2.2 is

$$\log m = \lambda_0 + \lambda_i^A + \lambda_j^B + \delta + \beta u_i u_j + \lambda^C + e.$$

In this equation, λ_0 is the intercept parameter, λ_i^A represents the parameters for the main effect of Rater A (rows), λ_j^B represents the parameters for the main effect of Rater B (columns), δ represents the parameters for the weights given to the cells in the main diagonal, $\beta u_i u_j$ represents the parameters for the linear by linear interaction, and λ^C represents the parameters for the covariates.

As was indicated above, each of these parameters can be part of a CFA base model, with the exception of the δ parameters. The δ parameters are introduced to devise a model of rater agreement. In the present exploratory context with focus on cell-wise testing, there is no modeling intent. Therefore, the δ parameters are not part of a CFA base model. It is the goal of CFA to identify those configurations (cells) that occur significantly more often (types) or less often (antitypes) than expected from some chance model. The base model is this chance model. The most complex CFA base model is therefore

$$\log m = \lambda_0 + \lambda_i^A + \lambda_j^B + \beta u_i u_j + \lambda^C + e.$$

The following sections present sample applications of CFA of rater agreement data. We begin with the most elementary base model, the main effect model.

3.2.1　CFA of Rater Agreement Data Using the Main Effect Base Model

In this section we re-analyze the data from Table 1.2. This re-analysis allows us to illustrate the statements that can be made based on CFA as compared to the application of coefficients and models of rater agreement. The data describe the agreement between two psychiatrists who re-evaluated the files of $N = 129$ clinically depressed inpatients. The psychiatrists evaluated the severity of the patients' depression. The rating categories were 1 = not depressed, 2 = mildly depressed, and 3 = clinically depressed. In the following exploratory configural analysis, we explore whether the two raters agree beyond chance in each of the three severity categories. From the earlier results, we know already that the agreement between these two raters is statistically significantly greater than could be expected from chance ($\hat{\kappa} = 0.375$; $\hat{\kappa}_n = 0.616$, and $\hat{ra} = 0.744$). In addition, we know that the equal weight agreement model parameter δ does not make a significant contribution to the explanation of these data.

If the two psychiatrists agree beyond chance in each of the three rating categories, each of the diagonal cells constitutes a type. In addition, we anticipate that at least some of the off-diagonals cells constitute antitypes. In the following sections, we re-analyze the data from Table 1.2 using the main effect base model, that is, the model $\log m = \lambda_0 + \lambda_i^A + \lambda_j^B + e$. We use the normal approximation of the binomial test and the Bonferroni-adjusted $\alpha^* = 0.05/9 = 0.00556$. Table 3.1 displays results of CFA.

Table 3.1: **First Order CFA of the Cross-Classification of Two Psychiatrists' Ratings (data from Table 1.2)**

Psychiatrist	Frequencies		Test Statistics		Type/ Antitype?
AB	observed	expected	z	p	
11	11	2.98	4.705	$< \alpha^*$	T
12	2	3.22	-0.691	.2449	
13	19	25.80	-1.496	.0673	
21	1	0.65	0.433	.3324	
22	3	0.71	2.739	.0031	T
23	3	5.64	-1.138	.1276	
31	0	8.37	-2.992	.0014	A
32	8	9.07	-0.368	.3563	
33	82	72.56	1.676	.0469	

[a]the expression $< \alpha^*$ indicates that the tail probability is smaller than can be expressed with four decimals.

The only antitype is constituted by Cell 31. From the base model, it was expected that the second psychiatrist would diagnose over 8 patients as not depressed that the first psychiatrist had diagnosed as clinically depressed.

However, there was not a single incidence of this disagreement pattern.

These results confirm the results obtained with Cohen's κ and the equal weight agreement model first by replicating the finding that the diagonal cells stand out. Both the largest number of agreements and all of the agreement that goes beyond chance can be found in the diagonal cells. However, CFA identifies two additional characteristics of the data. First, it shows that although Cell 33 contains the largest number of agreements, this number does not exceed the number expected from the base model. Thus, the diagonal cells differ greatly in their characteristics.

We conclude that Cells 11 and 22 on one side, and Cell 33 on the other reflect different characteristics of agreement data. Cells 11 and 22 contain frequencies that are significantly larger than expected from the base model. These are the instances in which agreement is *surprisingly strong*. In contrast, although Cell 33 contains the largest frequency, it is within expectation. Thus, the first characteristic is that agreement can be *greater than expected* (or *less than expected*). Coefficient κ and CFA are both sensitive to this characteristic. However, whereas κ aggregates over the agreement cells, CFA examines these cells individually. The second characteristic is that agreement can be highly frequent with or without exceeding an expected value. The coefficient of raw agreement is sensitive to this data characteristic. The main effect-based version of CFA discussed in this section and κ are sensitive to this characteristic only if this large frequency exceeds the expected frequency. This applies accordingly to the case in which the observed frequency is smaller than the expected frequency. In addition, this also applies to the disagreement cells. The next section introduces *zero order CFA*, a variant that uses the same base model as Brennan and Prediger's (1981) $κ_n$.

The performance of the equal weight agreement model on these data suggested that the weights might differ. The location of the difference and the specific and differential characteristics of the cells in the diagonal were identified using CFA. In addition, CFA allowed one to show that one particular disagreement pattern, the one in Cell 31, occurred significantly less often than expected from the base model. Readers are invited to confirm that the α protection procedure proposed by Hommel et al. (1985) would not have led to a different pattern of types and antitypes.

3.2.2   Zero Order CFA of Agreement Tables

As was discussed in Section 1.3 of this book, it is one of the criticisms of Cohen's κ that the measure evaluates *deviations from independence*, that is, *agreement beyond chance*, in the main diagonal of an agreement table instead of (relative) frequency of agreement. As a consequence if this characteristic, κ is considered *prevalence-dependent* (Guggenmoos-Holzmann, 1995). That is, κ can be low and suggest non-significant agreement beyond chance, even if the percentage of agreement is high. Therefore, Brennan and Prediger (1981) proposed using the no-effect base model instead of the main effect base model. The resulting coefficient, κ_n, does not suffer from these characteristics. It is sensitive to both main effects and interactions.

An analogous discussion can be had for the exploratory CFA of rater agreement, when performed under the main effect model illustrated in the last section. When the main effect base model is employed, CFA is sensitive only to interactions in a cross-classification. In other words types and antitypes of agreement and disagreement surface only if deviations occur after the main effects are taken into account. Consequently, it can happen that large frequencies fail to constitute types and small frequencies fail to constitute antitypes.

Consider, for example, Table 3.1 in Section 3.2.1. In this table, the largest observed frequency was 82, in Cell 33. This frequency did not deviate enough from the expected frequency that had been estimated under the main effect model to constitute an agreement type. Still, the raters agreed just in category 3 in 63.66% of all judgements in the table. Accordingly, the second smallest observed frequency in Table 3.1, a 1 for Cell 21, failed to constitute an antitype. (The smallest frequency, the 0 in Cell 31, did constitute an antitype.)

Thus, researchers may be interested in identifying cells as types and antitypes of agreement and disagreement when a null model is employed, that is, when main effects are not taken into account. Such a null model, in the context of CFA termed *zero order CFA base model*, takes no information into account that goes beyond the sample size. Thus, the model is $\log m = 1\lambda + e$. This model has a column vector of 1s for a design matrix and there is only one parameter that needs to be estimated, the intercept parameter. The estimated expected cell frequencies reflect a uniform distribution, that is, they are calculated as the sample size over the number of cells in the table. Deviations from these expected cell frequencies can occur because of the existence of main effects, because of the existence of an interaction, or both. Main effects suggest that raters use the rating categories at unequal rates. An interaction exists if ratings made by one rater carry information about the ratings made by the other rater, that is, when there is an association between two raters' judgements.

Data example. To illustrate the application of zero order CFA to rater agreement tables and to compare zero order CFA with first order CFA, we now re-analyze the data from Table 3.1. These data describe the agreement between two psychiatrists who rate the depression of 129 patients on a 3-point scale with 1 indicating 'not depressed.' To create comparable results, we again use the normal approximation of the binomial test and the Bonferroni-adjusted $\alpha* = 0.00556$. The base model for this zero order CFA is log $m = 1\lambda + e$. Table 3.2 displays the results.

Table 3.2:   Zero Order CFA of the Cross-Classification of Two Psychiatrists' Ratings (data from Table 1.2)

Psychiatrist	Frequencies		Test statistics		Type/ Antitype?
AB	observed	expected	z	p^a	
11	11	14.33	-0.934	.1752	
12	2	14.33	-3.455	.0003	A
13	19	14.33	1.307	.0955	
21	1	14.33	-3.735	$< \alpha*$	A
22	3	14.33	-3.175	.0007	A
23	3	14.33	-3.175	.0007	A
31	0	14.33	-4.016	$< \alpha*$	A
32	8	14.33	-1.774	.0380	
33	82	14.33	18.957	$< \alpha*$	T

[a] the expression $< \alpha*$ indicates that the tail probability is smaller than can be expressed with four decimals.

The overall goodness-of-fit for the zero order CFA base model for the data in Table 3.2 is LR-$X^2 = 249.62$ ($df = 8$; $p < 0.01$). Thus, this model describes the observed frequency distribution significantly worse than the main effect model used for Table 3.1 ($\Delta X^2 = 210.59$; $\Delta df = 4$; $p < 0.01$). The two models differ only in that the first order model did take the main effects into account whereas the zero order model did not. We thus learn that the main effects explain a large part of the variability in this agreement table. This does not come as a surprise, considering the marginal frequency distributions which reflect the psychiatrists' unequal use of the three rating categories. We observe that the Psychiatrist A used the first category 32 times, the second 7 times, and the third 90 times. The Psychiatrist B used the first, second, and third categories 12, 13, and 104 times, respectively.

Table 3.2 shows that zero order CFA identifies five antitypes and one type. As is plausible for agreement tables, the antitypes mostly suggest that disagreement is observed less often than expected. One of the antitypes, however, stands out. This antitype is constituted by Cell 22, an *agreement cell*. The two psychiatrists jointly diagnosed three patients' records as mildly depressed. From the null model, this was expected to occur over 14 times. We note that the two psychiatrists not only use this category rather infrequently, they also agree less often than expected in this middle category. Table 3.1 shows, that the category mildly depressed forms a type instead of an antitype when the main effects are taken into account. If the information about the uneven use of diagnostic categories is taken into account, one would not expect over 14 cases for Cell 22 but less than one, and the observed two are then significantly more than expected.

In more general terms, this example illustrates that the base models of CFA take different amounts of information into account when they estimate the expected cell frequencies. Therefore, the expected cell frequencies vary widely depending on the base model that is used. Typically, using more information moves the estimated expected cell frequencies closer to the observed cell frequencies. However, there are exceptions as can be seen when comparing Tables 3.1 and 3.2. For example, the z-score for Cell 12 in Table 3.1 (more information taken into account) is -1.496, whereas in Table 3.2 (less information taken into account) it is 1.307. More dramatically, the z-score for Cell 11 in Table 3.1 is 4.705, and in Table 3.2 it is -0.934. We see from these examples, that one has to expect different, even contradictory appraisals of cell frequencies if one uses different base models.

Before turning to analyzing rater agreement under consideration of the ordinal nature of rating variables, we ask what the reasons are for selecting first order versus zero order CFA for the exploration of rater agreement. Zero order CFA takes just the sample size into account when estimating expected cell frequencies. Thus, types and antitypes can emerge just because cell frequencies are large or small. The interpretation of such agreement types and antitypes refers to the (constant) expected cell frequencies. Types are thus agreement/disagreement patterns that occur significantly   more   often   than   average.   Antitypes   are agreement/disagreement patterns that occur significantly less often than average.

In contrast, types of agreement or disagreement in first order CFA indicate frequencies of agreement or disagreement that occur more often under consideration of the possibly different rates with which the raters use the rating categories. The same applies to antitypes. Obviously, Cohen's κ and first order CFA use the same base model. The agreement/disagreement types and antitypes of first order CFA are therefore also *prevalence-dependent* (Guggenmoos-Holzmann, 1995).

Thus, the question as to whether to use zero order or first order CFA for the exploration of agreement tables, finds a simple answer: Use both. Zero order CFA identifies the patterns that occurred significantly more often or less often than average. In zero order CFA, results are not prevalence-dependent. First order CFA finds the patterns that occur significantly more often or less often than expected under consideration of the differential rates with which raters use the rating categories.

3.2.3 CFA of Rater Agreement Data under Consideration of Linear-by-Linear Association for Ordinal Variables

In this section, we ask whether taking into account the ordinal nature of rating categories can be considered in the exploratory analysis of rater agreement data. Specifically, we now consider the base model

$$\log m = \lambda_0 + \lambda_i^A + \lambda_j^B + \beta u_i u_j + e.$$

This model is a special case of the general log-linear CFA base model discussed in Section 3.2. It sets the λ parameters for the covariates to zero. In addition, this model is hierarchically related to the most complex CFA base model in Section 3.2, the main effect base model in Section 3.2.1, and the zero order base model in Section 3.2.2.

To illustrate this model in exploratory research, we use the psychiatric data again. We ask whether taking into account the possibly ordinal nature of the three depression diagnoses changes the emerging pattern of types and antitypes. The design matrix for this base model appears in the following equation.

$$
\begin{bmatrix} \log m_{11} \\ \log m_{12} \\ \log m_{13} \\ \log m_{21} \\ \log m_{22} \\ \log m_{23} \\ \log m_{31} \\ \log m_{32} \\ \log m_{33} \end{bmatrix}
=
\begin{bmatrix}
1 & 1 & 0 & 1 & 0 & 1 \\
1 & 1 & 0 & 0 & 1 & 2 \\
1 & 1 & 0 & -1 & -1 & 3 \\
1 & 0 & 1 & 1 & 0 & 2 \\
1 & 0 & 1 & 0 & 1 & 4 \\
1 & 0 & 1 & -1 & -1 & 6 \\
1 & -1 & -1 & 1 & 0 & 3 \\
1 & -1 & -1 & 0 & 1 & 6 \\
1 & -1 & -1 & -1 & -1 & 9
\end{bmatrix}
\begin{bmatrix} \lambda_0 \\ \lambda_1^A \\ \lambda_2^A \\ \lambda_1^B \\ \lambda_2^B \\ \beta \end{bmatrix}
+
\begin{bmatrix} e_{11} \\ e_{12} \\ e_{13} \\ e_{21} \\ e_{22} \\ e_{23} \\ e_{31} \\ e_{32} \\ e_{33} \end{bmatrix}.
$$

This model is identical to the one given in Section 2.3.4, with the exception that there is neither a vector for a hypothesis concerning the main diagonal (last vector in X in Section 2.3.4) nor a parameter for this hypothesis (δ parameter).

Using this base model, we now perform a CFA of the data in Tables 1.2 and 3.1. We use the Pearson X^2 statistic for the cell-wise tests and the Bonferroni-adjusted $\alpha^* = 0.00556$. Table 3.3 displays the results from the CFA of these data. (Note that the results in Table 3.3 were created using SPSS. The program CFA2000 indicated estimation problems.)

Table 3.3:   **CFA of the Cross-Classification of Two Psychiatrists' Ratings (see Tables 2.2 and 4.1) under Consideration of the Ordinal Nature of the Diagnostic Categories**

| Cell | Frequencies | | Test Statistics | | Type/ |
AB	observed	expected	X^2	p	Antitype?
11	11	9.63	.195	.6589	
12	2	6.17	2.818	.0932	
13	19	16.20	.484	.4866	
					/ cont.

Cell	Frequencies		Test statistics		Type/
AB	observed	expected	X^2	p	Antitype?
21	1	0.62	.233	.6294	
22	3	0.91	4.800	.0285	
23	3	5.48	1.122	.2894	
31	0	1.75	1.750	.1859	
32	8	5.93	.723	.3953	
33	82	82.32	.001	.9719	

The addition of a covariate for a linear-by-linear association improved the main effect base model ($\Delta X^2 = 25.86$; $\Delta df = 1$; $p < 0.01$). However, the model fails to describe the data well, overall (LR-$X^2 = 13.17$; $df = 3$; $p = 0.0043$). Still, taking into account the ordinal nature of the diagnostic categories led to expected cell frequencies that are much closer to the observed cell frequencies than considering the diagnostic categories nominal level. The discrepancies are distributed such that no types or antitypes emerge. None of the cell-wise discrepancies is large enough to constitute a type or an antitype.

The result that taking into account the ordinal nature of variables reduces the chances for types and antitypes to emerge, can be generalized. Whenever additional information is included in a log-linear model or a CFA base model, the resulting expected cell frequencies are typically closer to the observed cell frequencies than without this information. In the present context of exploring rater agreement, additional information can come in two forms. The first is the linear-by-linear interaction included in the base model in the present section. The second is the form of continuous covariates. Thus, in most instances, using additional information leads to fewer types and antitypes (for exceptions see Glück & von Eye, 2000).

3.2.4 Using Categorical Covariates in CFA

As was illustrated in Section 2.3.3.1, taking into account categorical covariates often implies an unfolding of a cross-classification such that the cross-classification is created separately for each category of the covariate.

Tables 2.5 and 2.6 (Section 2.3.3.1) illustrate this unfolding. Often, a categorical covariate is considered a stratification variable. In the analysis of rater agreement, the question as to whether raters agree beyond chance is differentiated and one asks whether raters' agreement is (1) beyond chance and (2) the same in each stratum.

In the exploratory analysis of stratified rater agreement, a number of base models can be considered. The simplest base model, the main effect model of no variable interactions, is most appropriate when there exist no hypotheses about reasons for particular patterns of agreement or disagreement. If one hypothesizes in addition, that two raters' agreement-disagreement patterns are invariant across strata, the association between the two raters can be taken into account. The resulting types and antitypes will then indicate the configurations of rating categories in which the raters differentiate between the strata. The following data example illustrates both of these base models.

Data example. In the following example, we re-analyze the data from Section 2.3.3.1. A sample of 182 individuals rated the concreteness (1) abstractness (2) of proverbs and sentences. Stratification was by gender with 1 = females and 2 = males. The ratings of two proverbs are compared across the two gender groups. The observed frequencies appeared in Table 2.7, above.

We now subject the 2 x 2 x 2 cross-classification of Gender (G), Proverb 1 (P1), and Proverb 2 (P2) to exploratory CFA. We use the Pearson X^2 test, and Hommel et al.'s (1985) procedure for α protection. We consider two base models. The first is the main effect model $\log m = \lambda_0 + \lambda_i^G + \lambda_j^{P1} + \lambda_k^{P2} + e$, that is, the model of no interactions. Types and antitypes can emerge from this model because of any interaction among the three variables. The gender groups differ if types and antitypes appear for one group but not the other. However, types and antitypes can emerge for reasons other than gender differences, for instance, the association between P1 and P2. This possibility can make the interpretation of types and antitypes less than clear-cut. The second base model considered here, $\log m = \lambda_0 + \lambda_i^G + \lambda_j^{P1} + \lambda_k^{P2} + \lambda_{jk}^{P1,P2} + e$, proposes that, there is no association between rating of proverbs and gender. All three associations between gender and proverbs, that is G x P1, G x P2, and G x P1 x P2, are set to zero. Types and antitypes that emerge thus suggest that at least one of these associations exists.

The design matrix for the second base model is

$$X = \begin{bmatrix} 1 & 1 & 1 & 1 & 1 \\ 1 & 1 & 1 & -1 & -1 \\ 1 & 1 & -1 & 1 & -1 \\ 1 & 1 & -1 & -1 & 1 \\ 1 & -1 & 1 & 1 & 1 \\ 1 & -1 & 1 & -1 & -1 \\ 1 & -1 & -1 & 1 & -1 \\ 1 & -1 & -1 & -1 & 1 \end{bmatrix}.$$

The first column in this matrix contains the constant scores. The following three columns contain the vectors for the main effects of G, P1, and P2, in that order. The last column contains the vector for the P1 x P2 interaction. Note again that this matrix does not contain any vector for δ parameters. These are not part of CFA base models (cf. Section 2.3.3.1). The design matrix for the first base model considered here, that is, the main effect model, contains only the first four column vectors of X. The results of the CFA under the main effect model appear in Table 3.4.

Table 3.4:   **CFA of the Cross-Classification of Gender (G), Proverb 1 (P1), Proverb 2 (P2); Main Effect Base Model**

Configuration	Frequencies		Test statistics		Type/
G P1 P2	observed	expected	X^2	p	Antitype?
111	20	11.27	6.77	.0093	T
112	23	33.31	3.19	.0740	
121	8	22.35	9.21	.0024	A
122	82	66.07	3.84	.0500	
211	12	4.15	14.84	.0001	T
212	6	12.27	3.21	.0734	
221	6	8.23	0.61	.4363	/ cont.

| Configuration | Frequencies | | Test statistics | | Type/ |
G P1 P2	observed	expected	X^2	p	Antitype?
212	6	12.27	3.21	.0734	
221	6	8.23	0.61	.4363	
222	25	24.34	0.02	.8941	

The overall goodness-of-fit of the base model is poor (LR-X^2 = 39.32; df = 4; p < 0.01). We thus can expect types and antitypes to emerge. The results in Table 3.4 indicate that two types and one antitype exist. The two types are rater-agreement types. They suggest that both the female (Type 111) and the male subjects (Type 211) agree beyond chance when they rate proverbs as concrete. The antitype (121) appears in the female sample only. It suggests that rating the first proverb as concrete and the second as abstract is significantly less likely than expected by chance. Eight respondents were observed showing this pattern, whereas over 22 had been expected.

We now ask whether taking into account the association between the two proverbs leads to expected cell frequencies that are closer to the observed frequencies than the main effect base model and, perhaps, to a different pattern of types and antitypes. If a different pattern emerges, the pattern found based on first order CFA must be the result of one of the interactions with gender discussed above. The design matrix for this model was given above, before Table 3.4. To make results comparable, we again protected the significance level α using the Hommel et al. (1985) procedure, and we employed the Pearson X^2 test. Table 3.5 displays the results of this CFA.

The overall goodness-of-fit of this base model is excellent (LR-X^2 = 4.66; df = 3; p = 0.18). This model improves the main effect base model significantly (ΔX^2 = 34.66; df = 1; p < 0.01). In addition, because of the good fit, we cannot expect types and antitypes to emerge. Table 3.5 shows that not a single type or antitype emerged, in neither sample. We thus conclude that there exist no gender differences in the evaluation of the two proverbs. The two types and the sole antitype in the main effect-only CFA in Table 3.4 thus emerged only because the association between the two proverbs and gender exists but was not part of the base model. There are no gender differences that CFA can detect.

Table 3.5:   CFA of the Cross-Classification of Gender (G), Proverb 1 (P1), Proverb 2 (P2); No-Gender Association Base Model

Configuration	Frequencies		Test Statistics		Type/ Antitype?
G P1 P2	observed	expected	X^2	p	
111	20	23.39	0.49	.4840	
112	23	21.19	0.15	.6946	
121	8	10.23	0.49	.4855	
122	82	78.19	0.19	.6668	
211	12	8.62	1.33	.2489	
212	6	7.81	0.42	.5177	
221	6	3.77	1.32	.2505	
222	25	28.81	0.50	.4781	

3.3   Fusing Explanatory and Exploratory Research: Groups of Types

Thus far in this book, CFA focused on individual cells, the log-linear models focused on particular hypotheses, and κ focused on all agreement cells. In this section, we discuss application of CFA methods to groups of cells (see Stouffer, Suchman, DeVinney, Star, & Williams, 1949; for a discussion and extension see Darlington & Hayes, 2000; for an application within CFA see von Eye, 2002a). The general task is one that can be accomplished with *tests of combined significance*, the so-called *probability poolers*. The purpose of tests of combined significance in the present context of evaluation of rater agreement is to test whether, in a selection of diagonal cells, there is the desired effect, that is, agreement better than chance. (Later, in Section 3.5.2, we show how to apply these methods to the analysis of disagreement cells.)

There are specific instances, in which one needs tests of combined significance, although log-linear models and such coefficients as κ already operate at the aggregate level. However, there are instances in which probability poolers are the only choice. Consider the following two examples. First, a researcher finds a possibly strong yet non-significant κ, and suspects that agreement nevertheless is beyond chance in a number of categories. In this situation, the researcher can employ tests of combined significance to test this hypothesis for the categories under scrutiny. Second, there may be a situation in which particular categories are more important than others, for example, because consequences are more severe. For instance, categories may result from cut-offs for accepting or rejecting of candidates, articles, or proposals. In these situations, it may be of importance that raters agree in particular in the critical categories. The tests of combined significance allow one to evaluate rater agreement in these categories.

Stouffer's Z combines k probabilities in the following way. Consider k tests of the same null hypothesis, in different, independent data. Let z_i be the z-score of the ith test, for $i = 1, ..., k$. Then, the combined z-score of these k individual probabilities is

$$Z_{Stouffer} = \frac{\sum_{i=1}^{k} z_i}{\sqrt{k}} .$$

Under the null hypothesis, the Z-statistic is normally distributed if the individual z_i scores are independent of each other. The Z-score itself can be compared to the critical values for any α of the standard normal distribution.

In the application of tests of combined significance, we proceed in three steps:

(1)   either estimate probabilities p_{ii} for all diagonal cells and transform them into z_{ii}-scores, or estimate the z_{ii} scores directly for all cells of interest; either option can be performed using CFA or residual analysis in log-linear modeling;

(2)   select the rating categories to be included in the test of combined significance; and

(3)   calculate $Z_{Stouffer}$ for the selected cells and determine whether the selected cells in combination suggest significant rater agreement beyond chance.

These steps can accordingly be performed if the researchers are interested in particular patterns of disagreement (see Section 3.5.2).

Data example. For the following example, we use the data from Table 3.4 (see also Section 2.3.3.1). A sample of 182 individuals rated the concreteness (1) - abstractness (2) of proverbs and sentences. Stratification was by gender with 1 = females and 2 = males. The ratings of two proverbs are compared across the two gender groups. The raw frequencies of the 2 x 2 x 2 cross-classification of Gender (G), Proverb 1 (P1), and Proverb 2 (P2) appear in Tables 2.7 and 3.3, above.

The exploratory, configural approach to evaluating rater agreement had suggested the existence of two types, constituted by Cells 111 and 211, and one antitype, constituted by Cell 121. Cells 122 and 222 failed to constitute types. We now ask, whether the composite of the Cells 111, 122, 211, and 222 supports the hypothesis, that, in all these instances, rater agreement is better than chance. These are the cells in the two main diagonals of the two gender strata. Proceeding in the three steps outlined above, we obtain from the fifth column of Table 3.4 the probabilities of these four cells which we can transform into z-scores. (We could also have taken the X^2-scores from the fourth column, and then summed the square roots of the X^2-scores to obtain $Z_{Stouffer}$). Table 3.6 summarizes the results of the calculations for the test of combined significance.

Inserting the sum of the z-scores into the formula for Stouffer's Z yields $Z_{Stouffer} = \dfrac{8.9633}{\sqrt{4}} = 4.4817$ with $p < 0.01$. We thus can conclude that agreement in the composite of the four cells in the 2 x 2 x 2 cross-classification of Gender, Proverb 1, and Proverb 2 is greater than could be expected based on chance.

Inserting the sum of the z-scores into the Z formula yields $Z_{Stouffer} = \dfrac{8.9633}{\sqrt{4}} = 4.4817$ and $p < 0.01$. We thus conclude that the agreement in the composite of the four cells of which, individually, only two constituted types (see Table 3.4), is greater than could be expected based on chance.

We now ask whether agreement in the composite of the two cells that contain the majority of the judgements but did not constitute types of agreement is better than chance. These are the two cells 122 and 222. The sum of the z-scores for these two cells is $1.6449 + 1.2459 = 2.8908$. Inserting into the Z formula yields $Z_{stouffer} = 2.8908/\sqrt{2} = 2.0441$ with $p = 0.0205$. We thus conclude that the composite of those two cells, that, individually, do not constitute types, suggests agreement beyond chance.

Table 3.6:   Combining the Significance of Cells 111, 122, 211, and 222 from Table 3.4

Cell	p	z
111	.0093	2.3535
122	.0500	1.6449
211	.0001	3.7190
222	.8936	1.2459
Sum of z-scores		8.9633

3.4   Exploring the Agreement among Three Raters

When exploring the agreement and disagreement among three or more raters, one typically crosses the ratings provided by the raters with each other. For example, if m raters evaluate the same objects, one can cross the ratings to form an $I^m = I \times I \times I \times \dots$ contingency table. An example of such a table appeared in Table 2.15, in Section 2.4.1.1.

A CFA of such a contingency table allows researchers to identify those agreement cells in which two or more raters agree/disagree beyond chance, and those disagreement cells, that contain significantly more/fewer judgements than expected based on chance. It is important to realize that a three- or higher-dimensional cross-classification of raters' judgements contains various kinds of agreement cells. Specifically, there are the agreement cells for pairs of raters, triplets of raters, and so on. If researchers are interested in the agreement of subsets of raters, they can use the Stouffer's Z (see Section 3.3) to determine whether there is agreement beyond chance.

To illustrate, consider the 3 x 3 x 3 cross-classification in Table 2.15. This table contains two kinds of agreement cells, agreement cells (1) for pairs of raters and (2) for the triplet of raters. The agreement cells for the three pairs of raters have subscripts *ii.*, *i.i*, and *.ii* (the corresponding cells are identified in the last three columns of the design matrix in Section 2.4.1.1), the agreement cells for the triplet of raters have subscripts *iii*.

The most important CFA base model for the exploration of the agreement among three or more raters is the main effect model which proposes that the raters' judgements are independent. Types in agreement cells will then suggest that raters agree beyond chance. Antitypes in disagreement cells suggest that particular patterns of disagreement occur less often than expected based on chance. Types in disagreement cells and antitypes in agreement cells make the researcher worry.

Data example. In the following example, we re-analyze the data in Table 2.15. Three psychiatrists evaluated the depression diagnoses of 163 patients. They used the three categories 1 = not depressed, 2 = mildly depressed, and 3 = clinically depressed. We now analyze these data using CFA under the main effect base model $\log m = \lambda_0 + \lambda_i^A + \lambda_j^B + \lambda_k^C + e$, the Bonferroni-adjusted $\alpha^* = 0.00185$, and, because of the small sample size, the binomial test. Results appear in Table 3.7.

Table 3.7:   CFA of the Data in Table 3.6 (z-scores given only for the cells used for the subsequent analyses of composite types and antitypes)

| Configuration | Frequencies | | p from Binomial | Type/ | |
ABC	observed	expected	tests	Antitype?	z
111	4	.271	.0002	T	3.5746
112	3	.422	.0090		2.3656
113	6	4.215	.2477		0.6817
121	2	.244	.0252		1.9566
122	1	.379	.3160		
123	3	3.794	.4728		
131	2	1.694	.5059		0.0148
132	2	2.635	.5085		/ cont.

| Configuration | Frequencies | | p from Binomial tests | Type/ Antitype? | z |
ABC	observed	expected			
133	17	26.346	.0252		
211	0	.068	.9345		1.5102
212	1	.105	.1001		
213	2	1.054	.2841		
221	1	.061	.0592		
222	1	.095	.0905		
223	1	.948	.6137		
231	0	.423	.6544		
232	0	.659	.5169		
233	4	6.587	.2084		
311	0	.766	.4642		0.0899
312	1	1.191	.6657		
313	3	11.909	.0019		
321	0	.689	.5013		
322	1	1.072	.7093		
323	8	10.718	.2492		
331	0	4.785	.0078		
332	4	7.443	.1303		
333	96	74.429	.0005	T	3.3073

The LR-X^2 = 75.10 (df = 20; p < 0.01) indicates that the fit of the CFA base model is poor. We thus can expect types and antitypes to emerge. Table 3.7 shows two types. The first type is constituted by Cell 111. It suggests that the three psychiatrists agree beyond chance in their diagnoses of patients that are not depressed. The second type is constituted by Cell 333. It suggests that the three psychiatrists agree beyond chance in their diagnoses of patients that are clinically depressed. We thus conclude that the psychiatrists agree in the two extreme categories. It also seems that the psychiatrists did not make much use of the intermediate category. Only one patient was diagnosed as mildly depressed by all three raters. Finally, none of the disagreement cells constituted an antitype. Considering the small frequencies, this does not come as a surprise (Indurkhya & von Eye, 2000; von Eye, 2002b).

We now ask whether pairs of the three psychiatrists agree beyond chance. This question cannot be answered just from the CFA table, because the agreement of pairs of raters in individual configurations is split in three cells. For example, if one asks whether the raters A and B agree in their ratings of non-depressed patients, one has to look at Cells 111, 112, and 113. The composite of the ratings in these cells provides information about the agreement of rater A and rater B in Category 1.

To answer this question, we transform the probabilities of Configurations 111, 112, and 113 into z-scores (the z-scores for the following calculations are provided in Table 4.6), calculate the Stouffer Z (see Section 3.3) and obtain $Z_{Stouffer} = (3.5746 + 2.3656 + 0.6817)/\sqrt{3} = 3.8232$ with $p < 0.01$. We thus conclude that psychiatrists A and B agree beyond chance in their diagnoses of patients as not depressed.

Asking whether this holds true for the pairs A and C as well as B and C, we calculate for A and C $Z_{Stouffer} = (3.5746 + 1.9566 + 0.0148)/\sqrt{3} = 3.2020$ with $p < 0.01$. We thus conclude that psychiatrists A and C also agree beyond chance in their diagnoses of patients as not depressed. For psychiatrist pair B and C we obtain $Z_{Stouffer} = (3.5746 + 1.5102 + 0.0899)/\sqrt{3} = 2.9876$ with $p = 0.001$. We conclude that psychiatrists B and C also agree beyond chance in their diagnoses of patients as not depressed. Readers are invited to determine whether the three pairs of psychiatrists also agree beyond chance in their diagnoses of patients as mildly depressed and in their diagnoses of patients as clinically depressed.

3.5   What Else Is Going on in the Table: Blanking out Agreement Cells

In spite of the occasional counterexamples presented in various tables here in this text (see, e.g., Table 3.3), most agreement tables suggest solid agreement among raters. In addition, in most tables, the agreement cells, that is, the cells in the main diagonal of the agreement table are the ones with the largest observed frequencies. Still, one is often interested in finding out what is going on in the disagreement cells. Is there more disagreement than expected for particular patterns of judgements? Is there less disagreement than expected for other patterns of judgements? Is disagreement as expected for patterns of judgements?

This section discusses the analysis of disagreement cells. There are three ways in which disagreement cells can be analyzed using the methods presented in this text. First, using CFA, one can search for types or antitypes of disagreement in the complete table. This approach is discussed in Sections 3.2 and 3.3 and will, therefore, not be repeated here. A second approach involves blanking out the agreement cells first and then performing CFA. A third approach involves specifying a set of cells that are of particular interest and then analyzing them using Stouffer's Z, also after blanking out the agreement cells. The latter two approaches are discussed in this section. We begin with CFA of tables with blanked-out agreement cells.

3.5.1 CFA of Disagreement Cells

In this section, we propose *blanking out* the agreement cells of an agreement cross-classification and to then perform CFA on the disagreement cells only. With *blanking out*, we mean excluding cells from analysis. There are two reasons for blanking out agreement cells for the analysis of disagreement cells. First, agreement cells may belong to a different population of decisions than disagreements. Second, if the agreement cells carry the association in a cross-classification, the frequency distribution in the disagreement cells should be as predicted by the base model, and the frame of reference changes. For the analysis of disagreement cells, the reference population is the population of judgements, after blanking out the agreements. To illustrate, consider the agreement cross-classification that results when two raters use three categories for their judgements (from Table 1.1).

The shaded cells in this cross-classification, they contain the observed frequencies m_{ii}, are the agreement cells. Blanking these cells out yields a cross-classification as given in Table 3.9.

Table 3.8:   Cross-Classification of Two Raters' Judgements

		Rater B Rating Categories		
		1	2	3
Rater A Rating Categories	1	m_{11}	m_{12}	m_{13}
	2	m_{21}	m_{22}	m_{23}
	3	m_{31}	m_{32}	m_{33}

Table 3.9:   Cross-Classification of Two Raters' Judgements after Blanking out the Agreement Cells

		Rater B Rating Categories		
		1	2	3
Rater A Rating Categories	1	-	m_{12}	m_{13}
	2	m_{21}	-	m_{23}
	3	m_{31}	m_{32}	-

As is well known (Bishop, Fienberg, & Holland, 1975), this table cannot be reduced to a 3 x 2 or a 2 x 3 table. The reason is that the estimation of expected cell frequencies from the marginals of such a reduced table would use incorrect row and column sums. Consider, for example the 'reduced' cross-classification in Table 3.10.

In the cross-classification given in Table 3.10, the column sums use too many and incorrect summands. Consider the first column. Based on Table 3.9, we know that the column sum for this table is $m_{21} + m_{31}$. However, Table 3.10 falsely suggests that this column sum is $m_{12} + m_{21} + m_{31}$. This applies accordingly to the second column sum (and to the row sums if the cross-classification is condensed to be of size 2 x 3).

Table 3.10:   (Incorrectly) Reducing the 3 x 3 Cross-Classification of Two Raters' Judgements to a 3 x 2 Cross-Classification, after Blanking out the Agreement Cells

		Rater B Rating Categories	
		1/2	2/3
Rater A	1	m_{12}	m_{13}
Rating	2	m_{21}	m_{23}
Categories	3	m_{31}	m_{32}

The model used for the estimation of expected frequencies in a cross-classification of the type illustrated in Table 3.9 is called a *log-linear model of quasi-independence*. It has the form

$$\log m = \lambda + \lambda_i^A + \lambda_j^B + \lambda_k^C + e,$$

where the first three terms on the right hand side of the equation are as before and the third term denotes the parameters estimated for the coding variables that indicate which cells are blanked out. In explicit form, the quasi-independence model for the cross-classification Table 3.9 is

$$
\begin{bmatrix} \log m_{11} \\ \log m_{12} \\ \log m_{13} \\ \log m_{21} \\ \log m_{22} \\ \log m_{23} \\ \log m_{31} \\ \log m_{32} \\ \log m_{33} \end{bmatrix}
=
\begin{bmatrix}
1 & 1 & 0 & 1 & 0 & 1 & 0 & 0 \\
1 & 1 & 0 & 0 & 1 & 0 & 0 & 0 \\
1 & 1 & 0 & -1 & -1 & 0 & 0 & 0 \\
1 & 0 & 1 & 1 & 0 & 0 & 0 & 0 \\
1 & 0 & 1 & 0 & 1 & 0 & 1 & 0 \\
1 & 0 & 1 & -1 & -1 & 0 & 0 & 0 \\
1 & -1 & -1 & 1 & 0 & 0 & 0 & 0 \\
1 & -1 & -1 & 0 & 1 & 0 & 0 & 0 \\
1 & -1 & -1 & -1 & -1 & 0 & 0 & 1
\end{bmatrix}
\begin{bmatrix} \lambda_0 \\ \lambda_1^A \\ \lambda_2^A \\ \lambda_1^B \\ \lambda_2^B \\ \lambda_1^C \\ \lambda_2^C \\ \lambda_3^C \end{bmatrix}
+
\begin{bmatrix} e_{11} \\ e_{12} \\ e_{13} \\ e_{21} \\ e_{22} \\ e_{23} \\ e_{31} \\ e_{32} \\ e_{33} \end{bmatrix}.
$$

In this equation, the first five columns of the design matrix, that is, the first matrix on the right hand side of the equation, are identical to what we know from the log-linear models of rater agreement (see, e.g., the model in Section 2.3.4). The following three column vectors specify which cells are blanked out from the process of estimating the expected cell frequencies. The first of these three vectors blanks out Cell 11, the second blanks out Cell 22, and the third blanks out Cell 33.

When cells are blanked out from consideration, the following three implications need to be considered. First, the expected frequencies for the blanked-out cells are left untouched in the estimation process. They are not considered part of the table that is freed for estimation. Second, because the blanking-out of cells reduces the number of cells in the table, there are also fewer degrees of freedom available to work with. The quasi-independence log-linear model for a 3 x 3 table has 1 degree of freedom. Third, and this is most important for the analysis of rater agreement, if the cells with the largest frequencies are blanked out, the sample size will be smaller and thus there will be less power to rejected a false model.

The idea of blanking out cells that are probably type-constituting has been proposed for use in CFA by Kieser and Victor (1999). The idea of analyzing cells with blanked-out cells in the context of modeling rater-disagreement has been discussed by Bishop et al. (1975). When following this strategy in the context of configural analysis, one assumes that (1) the blanked-out cells contain cases that belong to a different population because they deviate significantly from the base model. If these cases belong to a different population, they should not be used to estimate expected frequencies for the remaining cases. One assumes also (2), that after blanking out type-cells, the remaining cells follow the distribution specified in the base model. In the present context of exploring rater agreement, this assumption implies that, after blanking out the diagonal cells, the disagreement cells show a distribution as specified in the base model of rater independence. If this model must be rejected, there may be patterns of disagreement that need to be discussed.

When employed in the context of modeling rater agreement, the model of quasi-independence allows one to ask an interesting question. The question is whether disagreement is distributed as expected from the assumption of rater independence, when agreement is left out of consideration. If the model prevails, one can conclude that the deviations from independence in the complete cross-classification are solely due to the agreement between the two raters. Disagreement would then be random. If, however, the model is rejected, there may be a pattern of disagreement that also contradicts the assumption of rater independence. CFA is a method that allows one to identify where in the cross-classification disagreement occurred more often or less often than expected.

Data example. The data for the following example are taken from Agresti (1996; see Landis & Koch, 1977). Two neurologists, A and B, diagnosed 149 cases of multiple sclerosis. They used the four categories 1 = certain multiple sclerosis, 2 = probable multiple sclerosis, 3 = possible multiple sclerosis, and 4 = doubtful, unlikely, or definitely not multiple sclerosis. We now re-analyze these data using two CFA models. First, we employ the main effect CFA base model which takes marginal probabilities into account. Second, we use the quasi-independence model presented in this section for the exploration of possible disagreement patterns. For both CFA runs, we use the z-test. For the first model, we calculate the the Bonferroni-adjusted $\alpha^* = 0.05/16 = 0.003125$. For the second model, the adjusted α is $\alpha^* = 0.05/12 = 0.00417$. Table 3.11 displays the results for the analysis under the main effect base model.

Table 3.11: CFA of Neurological Diagnosis Data under the Main Effect Base Model

Configuration	Frequencies		Tests		Type/ Anti-type?
AB	observed	expected	z	$p(z)^a$	
11	38	24.81	2.65	.0040	
12	5	10.93	-1.79	.0365	
13	0	3.25	-1.80	.0357	
14	1	5.02	-1.79	.0364	
21	33	26.50	1.26	.1032	
22	11	11.67	-0.20	.4221	
23	3	3.47	-0.25	.4004	
24	0	5.36	-2.32	.0103	/ cont.

| Configuration | Frequencies | | Tests | | Type/ |
AB	observed	expected	z	$p(z)^a$	Anti-type?
31	10	19.73	-2.19	.0142	
32	14	8.69	1.80	.0359	
33	5	2.58	1.50	.0664	
34	6	3.99	1.00	.1576	
41	3	12.97	-2.77	.0028	A
42	7	5.71	0.54	.2949	
43	3	1.70	1.00	.1589	
44	10	2.62	4.55	$< \alpha^*$	T

^{a} "$< \alpha^*$" indicates that the tail probability is smaller than can be expressed with 4 decimals.

The results in Table 3.11 suggest that patients are well advised consulting a third neurologist. Agreement is relatively low ($\hat{ra} = 0.43$; readers are invited to calculate $\hat{\kappa}$ and test it for significance). In addition, the two neurologists seem to agree beyond chance only in those cases that most likely do not suffer from multiple sclerosis (type in Cell 44). There is no impressive pattern of disagreement either. The only antitype for Cell 41 suggests that the two neurologists disagree less often than chance in those cases in which Neurologist A finds multiple sclerosis very unlikely, whereas Neurologist B considers it certain. The overall LR-$X^2 = 69.16$ ($df = 9$; $p < 0.01$) had suggested that there may be types and antitypes. However, CFA showed that there are many sizeable discrepancies, but only two of these turned out large enough to be significant under Bonferroni-adjustment.

We now ask whether the many cases of disagreement show significant deviations from independence when the relatively few cases of agreement are blanked out. To answer this question, we perform CFA under a log-linear quasi-independence base model. Table 3.12 displays the results. Again, because the four agreement cells are blanked out, we perform 12 instead of 16 significance tests, and obtain $\alpha^* = 0.00417$.

Table 3.12: **CFA of Neurological Diagnosis Data under a Quasi-Independence Base Model**

| Configuration | Frequencies | | Tests | | Type/ Anti- |
AB	observed	expected	z	$p(z)$	type?
11	38	38	-	-	
12	5	4.69	0.15	.4423	
13	0	0.67	-0.82	.2072	
14	1	0.65	0.44	.3308	
21	33	27.29	1.09	.1370	
22	11	11	-	-	
23	3	4.42	-0.68	.2499	
24	0	4.30	-2.07	.0191	
31	10	13.06	-0.85	.1983	
32	14	14.88	-0.23	.4099	
33	5	5	-	-	
34	6	2.06	2.75	.0030	T
41	3	5.65	-1.12	.1325	
42	7	6.44	0.22	.4119	
43	3	0.95	2.18	.0146	
44	10	10	-	-	

The results in Table 3.12 suggest that only one disagreement type exists. It is the type constituted by Cell 34. These are the six cases that Neurologist A diagnoses as 'possible multiple sclerosis,' whereas Neurologist B considers them as unlikely. No other discrepancy is strong enough to emerge as type or antitype. The overall LR-X^2 = 22.05 (df = 5; p < 0.01) suggests that the quasi-independence model is significantly better than the main effect model ($\Delta X^2 = 47.12$; $\Delta df = 4$; $p < 0.01$). However, although it fails to stand by itself, only one type emerged. This type had been obscured by the presence of the agreement cells in Table 3.10. In addition, the antitype with pattern 4 1 that had emerged before blanking out the diagonal cells, has now disappeared. In the following section, we use Stouffer's Z to test hypotheses concerning possible patterns of disagreement.

3.5.2 Testing Hypotheses about Disagreement

The results of the analyses in the last section suggested that the two neurologists (1) do not agree to an impressive degree, and (2) CFA detects only a small number of types and antitypes. The reason for this lack of types and antitypes may be that there exist patterns of deviations that, taken together are significant. Each of these deviations, taken individually, may fail to be significant, in particular under the strict regime of α-protection in CFA. In the following paragraphs, we approach the data in Table 3.12 with two hypotheses. First, we ask whether deviations by just one scale point are more likely than chance. Second, we ask whether deviations by more than one scale point are less likely than chance. Both hypotheses are tested in a one-tailed fashion and after blanking out the agreement cells. The z-scores are therefore taken from Table 3.12.

To test the first hypothesis, we include Cells 12, 21, 23, 32, 34, and 43. Inserting into the formula for Stouffer's Z, we obtain

$$Z_{Stouffer} = \frac{0.15 + 1.09 - 0.68 - 0.23 + 2.75 + 2.18}{\sqrt{6}} = 2.147.$$

This Z-score has a tail probability of 0.016. We thus reject the null hypothesis and claim that indeed rater disagreement by just one scale point is more likely than chance.

To test the second hypothesis, we include Cells 13, 14, 24, 31, 41, and 42. inserting yields

$$Z_{Stouffer} = \frac{-0.82 + 0.44 - 2.07 - 0.85 - 1.12 + 0.22}{\sqrt{6}} - -1.715.$$

This Z-score is also significant ($p = 0.043$). We thus conclude, based on the usual significance threshold of $\alpha = 0.05$, that disagreement between these two neurologists by more than two points on the scale of severity of multiple sclerosis is less likely than chance.

3.6 Exercises

3-1.   Using the data in Table 1.6, run the zero-order and first-order CFA
        models. How many types and antitypes are identified by each
        model?   Judging from the number and location of types and
        antitypes, do these models appropriately capture the data?

3-2.   Using the data in Table 1.6, run two nested CFAs with covariates of
        pair-specific agreement among three raters, and absolute agreement
        among all three raters. How many types and antitypes are identified
        by each model? Compare all four CFA models produced so far.
        Which CFA model is best?

3-3.   Consider the following 3 x 3 Table in which the weight in a sample
        of adolescents is rated as 1 = Underweight, 2 = Normal, and 3 =
        Overweight by two independent observers. Run a first-order CFA
        with covariates to blank out the agreement cells. What are the
        expected frequencies for the agreement cells? How is this model
        called in log-linear model analysis?

First Observer	Second Observer			Row Sum
	1	2	3	
1	24	10	4	38
2	7	38	19	64
3	3	15	28	46
Column Sum	34	63	51	148

3-4.   The data by Furman, Simon, Shaffer, and Bouchey (2002) are
        presented in the following 2 x 3 x 3 configuration table where S
        indicates the stratum variable (1 = Relationship with parents, 2 =
        Relationship with friends), P indicates the relationship experienced
        prior to romantic partners (1 = Secure, 2 = Preoccupied, 3 =
        Dismissing), and R indicates the relationship style with romantic
        partners (1 = Secure, 2 = Preoccupied, 3 = Dismissing). First, run
        a first-order CFA and identify types and antitypes. Interpret types

and antitypes.

SPR	Observed Frequency
111	18
112	2
113	4
121	1
122	2
123	0
131	23
132	5
133	10
211	24
212	4
213	3
221	3
222	7
223	1
231	15
232	0
233	10

3-5.   Based on the first-order CFA results from the question 3-4, test whether having dismissing relationships with parents or friends but secure relationships with romantic partners is less likely than chance (cell configurations of 131 and 231, respectively). Use Stouffer's Z. Also test the opposite hypothesis that it is less likely than chance to have secure relationships with parents or friends but dismissing relationship with romantic partners among adolescents (cell configurations 113 and 213, respectively).

4. Correlation Structures

Thus far in this text and in most parts of the literature on methods for the assessment of rater agreement, the focus was on the agreement of two or more raters when using a series of categories, all of which implicitly being indicators of one and the same variable. Agreement was then expressed in terms of, for instance, percent of matches (raw agreement; main diagonal) or observed proportion of agreement as compared to expected proportion of agreement (κ and its variants). In real life, however, that is, outside of journal articles on methods of rater agreement, assessments and evaluations of objects, persons, or programs are typically performed using multiple variables and dimensions.

For example, before students are admitted to some university, they have to compile a number of indicators of their university-worthiness, including, for example, SAT scores, GPA scores, letters of recommendation, personal statements, and statements about participation in extra-curricular activities and community service. All this information and more is considered when admission decisions are made. Before submitting this information, prospective students ask friends, counselors, teachers, even relatives to look over their materials and give them advise on how to improve on content and presentation. When feedback is unequivocal and positive, materials are submitted.

In studies of human development and developmental psychopathology, a need for multiple behavioral measures via multiple sources has been documented (O'Connor & Rutter, 1996). For example, a child's disruptive behavior can be reported by many sources, including the child, mother, father, and teachers, all using the same questionnaire with common metric and variance. One common way to report convergence, or lack thereof, among multiple informants is via zero-order correlation coefficients. In the case of four informants, there could be six pair-wise correlation coefficients to report. A correlation coefficient in this context can be interpreted as the expected agreement in *relative standing*s of objects on a measure of random cases between two sources.

In this chapter, we introduce alternative ways to assess agreement among raters or multiple sources of information. First, we introduce the intraclass correlation coefficient (ICC) and different models. We also illustrate how the ICC is related to Pearson's (1901) correlation coefficient ρ, and an internal consistency measure, Cronbach's α. Second, we introduce a method to compare correlation structures.

4.1   Intraclass Correlation Coefficients

The intraclass correlation coefficient (ICC; Pearson, 1901) is a variance decomposition method to assess the portion of overall variance attributable to between-subject variability (Li & Li, 2003). The theoretical ICC formula for a population can be expressed as:

$$ICC = \frac{\sigma_B^2}{\sigma_B^2 + \sigma_W^2},$$

where σ_B^2 indicates the variance between cases (i.e., objects or targets), and σ_W^2 indicates the variance within cases. These two components cover the total variance of the ratings. Both components can be estimated using Analysis of Variance (ANOVA) methods.

Table 4.1 shows a typical data matrix. Cases are assumed to be selected randomly from a population of interest, and raters are assumed to share common metric and homogeneous variance (i.e., *intra*class variance). As long as the assumption of equal *intra*class variance is fulfilled, the ICC is not limited to rater agreement; it can also be used with repeated measures such as annual measurements of self-esteem during adolescence or related measures such as measurement of all family members on behavioral traits of a random sample of objects.

Table 4.1:   A Data Matrix

Case (i)	Rater (j)						
	1	2	3	·	·	·	k
1	y_{11}	y_{12}	y_{13}	·	·	·	y_{1k}
2	y_{21}	y_{22}	y_{23}	·	·	·	y_{2k}
3	y_{31}	y_{32}	y_{33}	·	·	·	y_{3k}
·	·	·	·	·	·	·	·
·	·	·	·	·	·	·	·
n	y_{n1}	y_{n2}	y_{n3}	·	·	·	y_{nk}

Several ICC models exist that differ in the way variance is decomposed (McGraw & Wong, 1996; Shrout & Fleiss, 1979; Wong & McGraw, 1999). Formulas for extended models are available in McGraw and Wong (1996) and Wong and McGraw (1999). In this section, we focus on the three modes and two types of ICCs that were illustrated by Shrout and Fleiss. They are easily computed using a general purpose software program. The file *COMPUTERILLUSTRATIONS 1* on the CD that comes with this text graphically illustrates steps to compute the ICC using SPSS.

First, one has to specify rater characteristics. As noted previously in all ICCs, cases are assumed to be selected randomly. Depending on rater characteristics, there are three major classes of intraclass correlation coefficients: One-way random, Two-way random, and Two-way mixed. If the ordering of raters is irrelevant, then the *one-way random* ICC is appropriate for the data. In the one-way random ICC model, raters can be different for different cases. Therefore, only one systematic source of variation exists, which is attributable to cases. The *two-way random* ICC is appropriate when each rater rated all cases and raters are a random selection from a population of interest. Here, rater variability is taken into account. The *two-way mixed* ICC is the proper choice when a group of raters is unique and cannot be replaced so that objects or cases are random but the raters are fixed. However, two-way mixed ICC cannot be generalized to different samples and the ICC sample estimate is calculated using the same calculation as two-way random ICCs, although population definitions of two-way fixed models are different than those of two-way random models.

Second, one has to determine whether the unit of analysis is a single observation or averaged observation (averaged rating for k^{th} judge, the average score for a nth case). In Table 4.1, if y_{ij} represents a score from a single observation, *Single Measure* ICCs should be applied and interpreted. On the other hand, if y_{ij} indicates a score from average observations, an *Average Measure* ICC is used.

Third and finally, we need to consider what constitutes agreement and disagreement. If disagreement is understood not only in terms of relative standings given to cases but also in absolute scores, then ICC *Absolute Agreement* is appropriate. If relative ratings among cases is the only thing that matters, then ICC *Consistency* is appropriate. Different raters may create the same rank-ordering of objects but using different standards. So raters may agree on the relative standing of objects (agreement in consistency) but not in absolute sense (agreement in scores as well). For example, ratings of 1, 2, 3 and ratings of 5, 6, 7 on the group of three cases will result in 1 for both consistency ICC and Pearson's correlation estimates, but in .111 and .200 for absolute agreement ICC single and average measures, respectively. Technical details follow below.

ICCs can be interpreted as the extent to which there is an agreement (consistency or absolute agreement) among raters when objects are randomly selected. The generalizibility coefficient and Cronbach's alpha are special cases of two-way random average score ICC with consistency definition of agreement. A generalizibility coefficient indicates the portion of variance due to experimental conditions that can be generalized. Cronbach's alpha indicates the portion of variance that is due to true traits without measurement error (i.e., consistency among measures). In essence, the ICC is the correlation between one rating (either a single rating or a mean of several ratings) on a case or object and another rating obtained on the same case or object. If the assumptions of common metric and homogeneous variance are fulfilled (i.e., ratings or measurements are of a single class), the single measure ICC/consistency estimates equal Pearson's correlation coefficient estimate. For example, ratings of 1, 2, 3 and ratings of 3, 6, 9 on the group of three cases will result in $r = 1$ but only .60 and .75 for consistency ICC single and average measures, respectively. This discrepancy between Pearson's r and the ICC can be attributed to unequal variance: the standard deviation of Rater 1 was 1.0, whereas the standard deviation of Rater 3 was 3.0. Unlike Pearson's r, the ICC assumes homogeneous variances, and is sensitive to violations. Table 4.2

summarizes these sample results.

Table 4.2:   A Comparison of ICC Consistency and Absolute Agreement, and Pearson's Correlation

Case	Raters 1 & 2		Raters 1 & 3		Raters 2 & 3	
	1	2	1	3	2	3
1	1	5	1	3	5	3
2	2	6	2	6	6	6
3	3	7	3	9	7	9
Mean (SD)	2 (1)	6 (1)	2 (1)	6 (3)	6 (1)	6 (3)
r	1		1		1	
ICC Consistency	1 (single) 1 (average)		.60 (single) .75 (average)		.60 (single) .75 (average)	
ICC Absolute Agreement	.11 (single) .20 (average)		.24 (single) .39 (average)		.69 (single) .82 (average)	

Data example. Table 4.3 is adapted from Shrout and Fleiss (1979). A glance at the table reveals that the four raters' rating on the same case differ substantially. On average, Case 5 received the highest rating across the four raters, followed by Cases 3, 1, 6, 4, and 2. In addition, it is clear that Rater 1 was most lenient of all raters and Rater 2 was most strict. Sources of variability of the 6 by 4 data matrix can be traced to two components. The ANOVA table shows that these two sources of variance: Between cases and within cases. Variability due to within-case differences can further be broken down to two components: variability due to raters and residuals unaccounted for.

Formulas to estimate population ICCs and estimates using the data in Table 4.3 are presented in Table 4.4. For illustration purposes, we assume that for each of ICC, the above-mentioned assumptions are fulfilled. Table 4.4 shows are several visible patterns. The ICC that focuses on absolute agreement has lower estimates than the ones that focus on consistency because it additionally takes mean differences among raters into account. Second, average measure ICCs are higher than single measure ICC estimates. Third, two-way random measures produce higher estimates than one-way random measures.

Table 4.3:   **Four Ratings on Six Cases (adapted from Shrout and Fleiss, 1979)**

Case	Rater 1	Rater 2	Rater 3	Rater 4
1	9	2	5	8
2	6	1	3	2
3	8	4	6	8
4	7	1	2	6
5	10	5	6	9
6	6	2	4	7
Mean	7.67	2.50	4.33	6.67
SD	1.63	1.64	1.63	2.50

Analysis of Variance

Source	SS	df	MS	F
Between cases (BC)	56.21	5	11.24	
Within cases (WC)	112.75	18	6.26	
Between measures (BM)	97.46	3	32.49	31.87
Residuals (E)	15.29	15	1.02	
Total	168.96	23	7.35	

Table 4.4:   Formulas to Estimate Population ICCs and Estimates

---

One-way random

Consistency

$$\text{Single score ICC} = \frac{MS_{BC} - MS_{WC}}{MS_{BC} + (k-1)MS_{WC}} = .166$$

$$\text{Average score ICC} = \frac{MS_{BC} - MS_{WC}}{MS_{BC}} = .443$$

Two-way random

Consistency

$$\text{Single score ICC} = \frac{MS_{BC} - MS_E}{MS_{BC} + (k-1)MS_E} = .715$$

$$\text{Average score ICC} = \frac{MS_{BC} - MS_E}{MS_{BC}} = \alpha = .909$$

Absolute
Agreement

$$\text{Single score ICC} = \frac{MS_{BC} - MS_E}{MS_{BC} + (k-1)MS_E + \frac{k}{n}(MS_{BM} - MS_E)} = .290$$

$$\text{Average score ICC} = \frac{MS_{BC} - MS_E}{MS_{BC} + \frac{1}{n}(MS_{BM} - MS_E)} = .620$$

Pearson's correlation coefficient estimates, rs, among Raters 1, 2, and 3 were identical to single measure ICC/consistency estimates to the 3rd decimal point: .745 (Raters 1 and 2), .725 (Raters 1 and 3), and .894 (Raters 2 and 3). However, correlations differed from ICC estimates when it involved Rater 4. Correlations between Rater 4 with the rest of raters were .750, .729, and .718 while single measure ICCs (Consistency) were .687, .669, and .657, respectively with Raters 1, 2, and 3. The discrepancy reflects that while the variance of Raters 1, 2, and 3 was approximately identical, Rater 4 had a bigger variance across the 6 rated cases, indicating that the ICC is sensitive to unequal variance across measurements and ratings.

The intraclass correlation coefficient also finds use in multilevel regression analysis as a measure of the proportion of the variance explained by the grouping structure in the population. Table 4.3 shows that four raters provide repeated or nested measures for each of six cases, a typical situation for multilevel regression analysis. Without additional explanatory variables, this analysis would be equivalent to an *intercept-only* or *fully unconditional* multilevel regression model, that is, a one-way ANOVA with random effects. At level 1, the i-th score of an individual, provided by the j-th rater can be explained as follows:

$$y_{ij} = \beta_{0j} + e_{ij} ,$$

where, at level 2,

$$\beta_{0j} = \gamma_{00} + \mu_{0j} ,$$

where β_{0j} indicates the mean score given by the j-th rater, and e_{ij}, the level 1 error, indicates the discrepancy between the real observation, y_{ij}, and the β_{0j}. At the second level, γ_{00} and μ_{0j} indicate the intercept (also called *grand mean*), and the discrepancy or second level error, respectively. When we put these two equations into one, we find that there are two separate error terms,

$$y_{ij} = \gamma_{00} + \mu_{0j} + e_{ij} .$$

The Intraclass Correlation Coefficient, ICC, is then calculated as the proportion of the second level variance relative to the total variance, or

$$ICC = \frac{\sigma^2_{\mu_0}}{\sigma^2_{\mu_0} + \sigma^2_e} .$$

Using the data in Table 4.3, we calculate an ICC estimate of 0.492 from the error variances of 3.575 at the first level and 3.465 at the second level. This estimate can be interpreted as the proportion of variance that the raters share in common.

4.2   Comparing Correlation Matrices Using LISREL

Researchers often collect information from various sources. For example, in a study on adolescent development Ohannessian, Lerner, Lerner, and von Eye (2000) compared adolescents' and their parents' perceptions of family functioning and adolescent self-competence. In this study, family functioning was measured using such variables as adaptability, cohesion, and adjustment. Adolescent self-competence was assessed in relation to such variables as academic, social and athletic competence, physical attractiveness, and conduct behavior. One question that was asked concerned the similarities of the adolescents' perceptions with both fathers' and mothers' perceptions. In a related study, Ohannessian et al. (1995) compared parents' and adolescents' perceptions of the adolescents' emotional adjustment. In these and similar studies, multiple variables are used, and it is asked whether agreement exists across all variables.

There are many ways to answer the question whether agreement exists across many variables for a sample of raters. For example, one can ask whether the variable means are the same for the raters. One can also ask whether the factor structure of the variables is invariant across rater groups. One can specify models that include hypotheses about both factor and means structures. One can specify path models and compare them across groups. At the level of individual correlations, one can ask whether corresponding correlations in two groups differ significantly from each other. There are other options.

Here, we focus on the structure of the correlations among manifest variables. We do not discuss factor structures. Nor do we discuss differences in pairs of correlations. Furthermore, we do not deal with questions that concern mean differences. These questions can be answered using analysis of variance techniques. Instead, we ask whether the correlation or covariance structures of manifest variables are invariant across two or more groups of raters.

Correlation structures can be compared using methods of structural equations modeling (Jöreskog & Sörbom, 1993; Kline, 1998; Pugesek, Tomer, & von Eye, 2003). In the following section, we introduce the methods needed to compare correlation structures. We use Jöreskog and Sörbom's LISREL notation (see Jöreskog & Sörbom, 1993).

Consider the situation in which G groups of raters rate a number of cases on several variables. For Group g, the correlation matrix (Phi) of these variables, aggregated across all raters in this group, is $\Phi^{(g)}$, with $g = 1, ..., G$. To test the hypothesis that the correlation matrices are invariant across the G groups, we specify

$$\Phi^{(1)} = \Phi^{(2)} = \dots = \Phi^{(G)}.$$

The correlation matrices Φ are of the ususal kind, with ones in the diagonal and correlations in the off-diagonals. The corresponding residual variance-covariance matrices are the Θ_δ-matrices (Theta$_{\text{delta}}$). When testing the above hypothesis, one can pursue a number of options. First, one can specify that the residual matrices be invariant also, that is,

$$\Theta_\delta^{(1)} = \Theta_\delta^{(2)} = \dots = \Theta_\delta^{(G)}.$$

The diagonal elements of the Θ_δ-matrices contain the residuals of the diagonals of the correlation matrices. If one specifies the Θ_δ-matrices to be diagonal matrices, covariations among residuals are supposed not to exist. If, however, off-diagonal elements of the Θ_δ-matrices are freed, covariations among residuals are made part of the model. In the present context, there are two options for freeing residual covariations. First, one can free the same off-diagonal elements of Θ_δ-matrices for each group. This procedure would test the hypothesis that the covariations are invariant across groups. Alternatively, one can free residuals in a group-specific way. This procedure would test the hypothesis of invariant correlation matrices with the proviso that there exist group-specific residual covariations.

For the model optimization procedure, all fit functions that are available for model fitting are available too. That is, one can select from generalized least squares (GL), maximum likelihood (ML), unweighted least squares (UL) and other fit functions. In multigroup situations as the present one, LISREL minimizes the fit function

$$F = \sum_{g=1}^{G} \frac{N_g}{N} F_g(S^{(g)}, \Sigma^{(g)}, W^{(g)}) ,$$

where F is any of the above fit functions, N_g is the sample size of Group g, and the total sample size is $N = \Sigma_g N_g$; $S^{(g)}$ and $\Sigma^{(g)}$ are the sample and the population correlation matrices for Group g, and $W^{(g)}$ is the weight matrix for Group g. In the following examples, we use no weights. Therefore, $W^{(g)}$ is the identity matrix for all g. All this applies accordingly if covariance matrices are used instead of correlation matrices.

The overall goodness-of-fit can be assessed using the χ^2-distributed statistic $(N - 1)F$ with $df = 0.5\ G\ d\ (d + 1) - t$, where d is the number of variables and t is the number of independent parameters estimated in all groups. Other goodness-of-fit indicators such as the root mean square error of approximation (RMSEA) also need to be considered for model appraisal.

   In addition to the overall goodness-of-fit indicators, LISREL produces group-specific indicators when ML is used (the information provided by LISREL depends on the fit function that is used). Thus, one can determine which of the G groups deviates the most from the model that was optimized taking all groups into account.

Data example. The following data example presents a re-analysis of data published by Ohannessian, Lerner, Lerner, and von Eye (1995). The authors report the correlations between 9 family functioning measures that had been presented to girls and boys in 74 families. The respondents were, on average, 13 years old when they responded to the instruments for a second time. These are the data analyzed here. Family Functioning was assessed in terms of Family Adjustment (FA), Family Cohesion (FC), and Family Adaptability (FAD). Each of these three dimensions was assessed in regard to the respondent (A), their mother (M), and their father (F). Thus, correlation matrices were calculated for the nine variables FAA, FAM, FAF, FCA, FCM, FCF, FADA, FADM, and FADF. One correlation matrix each was calculated for the girls and for the boys in the 74 families. We now ask whether the girls and the boys agree in their appraisals of family functioning at the level of correlations among manifest variable correlations. The correlation matrices are reproduced in Table 4.5.

Table 4.5:   Pearson Correlations among Family Functioning Measures for Girls (Above Diagonal) and Boys (Below Diagonal) of 74 Families

Measure	1	2	3	4	5	6	7	8	9
1. FAA	-	.30	.20	.63	.38	.03	.40	.40	.35
2. FAM	.26	-	.41	.14	.72	.40	.02	.26	.03
3. FAF	.07	.32	-	.21	.29	.60	-.03	.14	.11
4. FCA	.58	.24	.09	-	.07	.19	.56	.27	.32
5. FCM	.03	.35	.12	.26	-	.52	.02	.55	.08
6. FCF	-.05	.17	.51	.21	.33	-	.06	.25	.13
7. FADA	.29	.06	.03	.60	.29	.05	-	.25	.37
8. FADM	-.31	.13	.12	-.09	.22	.20	.09	-	.52
9. FADF	-.02	.02	.49	.01	.33	.36	.12	.49	-

We report results from two models. The first model is strict and posits first that the correlation matrices are invariant across the groups of female and male adolescent respondent. More specifically, the first model posits that

$$\Phi^{(1)} = \Phi^{(2)}.$$

In addition, the first model constrains the residual variance/covariance matrices to be invariant across the two groups also, that is,

$$\Theta_\delta^{(1)} = \Theta_\delta^{(2)}.$$

This model is rather restrictive. Therefore, we anticipate that modifications may be needed. In a first modification step, we will allow for group-specific covariances among residuals. In a next modification step, one can, if needed, free selected correlations from the constraint of being invariant across groups. If freeing such residual covariances and correlations does not lead us to an acceptable model, we declare that the girls and the boys on these families present different perspectives of family functioning. The following analyses were performed using ML in LISREL 8.53. The command files are presented in Section 5.6.

Results for Model 1

The following list contains the goodness-of-fit estimates that LISREL provides for the first overall model, that is, the model of invariant correlation matrices and residual variance-covariance matrices.

```
               Global Goodness of Fit Statistics

                     Degrees of Freedom = 45
           Minimum Fit Function Chi-Square = 116.33 (P = 0.00)
Normal Theory Weighted Least Squares Chi-Square = 93.20 (P = 0.00)
            Estimated Non-centrality Parameter (NCP) = 48.20
         90 Percent Confidence Interval for NCP = (24.34 ; 79.82)

                  Minimum Fit Function Value = 0.80
        Population Discrepancy Function Value (F0) = 0.35
         90 Percent Confidence Interval for F0 = (0.18 ; 0.58)
        Root Mean Square Error of Approximation (RMSEA) = 0.13
       90 Percent Confidence Interval for RMSEA = (0.089 ; 0.16)
         P-Value for Test of Close Fit (RMSEA < 0.05) = 0.038

              Expected Cross-Validation Index (ECVI) = 1.34
        90 Percent Confidence Interval for ECVI = (1.16 ; 1.57)
                  ECVI for Saturated Model = 0.66
                ECVI for Independence Model = 3.84

   Chi-Square for Independence Model with 72 Degrees of Freedom = 508.15
                     Independence AIC = 544.15
```

```
                   Model AIC = 183.20
               Saturated AIC = 180.00
            Independence CAIC = 616.10
                  Model CAIC = 363.07
              Saturated CAIC = 539.75

          Normed Fit Index (NFI) = 0.77
      Non-Normed Fit Index (NNFI) = 0.74
 Parsimony Normed Fit Index (PNFI) = 0.48
     Comparative Fit Index (CFI) = 0.84
     Incremental Fit Index (IFI) = 0.85
        Relative Fit Index (RFI) = 0.63

               Critical N (CN) = 88.80
```

The estimates in this list suggest a rather modest model - data fit. Both Chi-Square measures suggest significant model-data differences; the RMSEA is above the usual cut-off of 0.05 or even 0.08. The group of girls contributes 59.77% to the overall Chi-Squared and has a GFI = 0.86. The group of boys contributes the slightly smaller percentage of 40.23% to the overall Chi-Squared and has the slightly better GFI = 0.89. Clearly, the model represents the correlation matrix for neither group satisfactorily.

Thus, although this model is not really a catastrophe, there is ample room for improvement. We thus free residual covariances as indicated by the modification indices. After having freed four residual covariances in the group of the boys,[8] we arrive at an tenable model. The following list presents the overall goodness-of-fit information.

```
           Global Goodness of Fit Statistics

                Degrees of Freedom = 32
      Minimum Fit Function Chi-Square = 38.55 (P = 0.20)
 Normal Theory Weighted Least Squares Chi-Square = 36.77 (P = 0.26)
    Estimated Non-centrality Parameter (NCP) = 4.77
    90 Percent Confidence Interval for NCP = (0.0 ; 23.99)

            Minimum Fit Function Value = 0.26
    Population Discrepancy Function Value (F0) = 0.035
     90 Percent Confidence Interval for F0 = (0.0 ; 0.18)
   Root Mean Square Error of Approximation (RMSEA) = 0.047
   90 Percent Confidence Interval for RMSEA = (0.0 ; 0.10)
    P-Value for Test of Close Fit (RMSEA < 0.05) = 0.63

        Expected Cross-Validation Index (ECVI) = 1.12
     90 Percent Confidence Interval for ECVI = (1.08 ; 1.26)
             ECVI for Saturated Model = 0.66
           ECVI for Independence Model = 3.84

Chi-Square for Independence Model with 72 Degrees of Freedom = 508.15
```

---

[8] Details concerning the freed residual covariances are provided in Section 5.6, on the program specification of these two models.

```
      Independence AIC = 544.15
            Model AIC = 152.77
        Saturated AIC = 180.00
     Independence CAIC = 616.10
           Model CAIC = 384.61
       Saturated CAIC = 539.75

        Normed Fit Index (NFI) = 0.92
    Non-Normed Fit Index (NNFI) = 0.97
Parsimony Normed Fit Index (PNFI) = 0.41
    Comparative Fit Index (CFI) = 0.98
   Incremental Fit Index (IFI) = 0.99
      Relative Fit Index (RFI) = 0.83

           Critical N (CN) = 203.60
```

The modified model indicates no significant model - data discrepancies. Both Chi-Squared values are small. In addition, the RMSEA = 0.047 now is below the close fit threshold of 0.05, and it does not contradict the null hypothesis of close fit (RMSEA < 0.05; p = 0.63). As before, the two groups contribute unequal portions to the overall chi-Squared. In the group of girls, the Chi-Squared is 17.36, a 45.04% contribution to the overall Chi-Squared. The GFI for the girls is 0.95. In the group of boys, the Chi-Squared is 21.19, that is, 54.96% of the overall Chi-Squared. The GFI for the boys is 0.94. We thus conclude that this model is defensible. In addition, this model is significantly better than the first, the stricter model. We calculate for the minimum fit Chi-Squared the ΔX^2 = 77.78 (Δdf = 4; p < 0.01) and note that the improvement is significant.

From these two models, we conclude that the girls and the boys in the families in the Ohannessian et al. (1995) study provide information about family functioning that has identical correlation structures. The boys differ from the girls in that four residual covariances are needed to arrive at a tenable model - data correspondence.

4.3 Exercises

4-1.   The following artificial data contain ratings of six individuals by five judges. Assume that these five judges were selected randomly from a nine-judge panel. Estimate the intraclass correlation coefficient for the data, and verify that the estimate of Cronbach's alpha is equal to the average ICC Consistency estimate.

	Judge 1	Judge 2	Judge 3	Judge 4	Judge 5
Katie	1	2	2	2	2
Elise	2	1	1	3	4
Michelle	4	4	3	1	1
Jen	3	3	5	4	3
Mary	5	6	6	5	5
Diana	6	5	4	6	6

4-2.   The following artificial data contain the correlation matrix of nine disruptive kinds of behavior of children as rated by their fathers (n = 100, upper triangle) and mothers (n = 100, lower triangles). Using LISREL, test whether agreement exists between maternal and paternal observations of their child's disruptive behavior. In other words, test the equality of correlation structures Φ and Θ_δ between maternal and paternal reports. What are values of goodness-of-fit measures? Is there reasonable room for improvement of the model? What conclusion would you draw from the results?

	1	2	3	4	5	6	7	8	9
1	--	.467	.543	.460	.270	.345	.425	.222	.233
2	.496	--	.505	.342	.435	.395	.171	.338	.300
3	.424	.495	--	.366	.336	.555	.241	.285	.423

/ cont.

	1	2	3	4	5	6	7	8	9
4	.610	.320	.378	--	.436	.552	.628	.362	.485
5	.463	.465	.444	.441	--	.597	.265	.589	.499
6	.379	.499	.486	.567	.666	--	.403	.485	.699
7	.402	.221	.327	.557	.373	.365	--	.410	.553
8	.306	.481	.388	.424	.524	.414	.536	--	.664
9	.313	.325	.479	.406	.527	.662	.604	.614	--

5.   Computer Applications

This chapter is concerned with computational issues. It is demonstrated how to calculate κ and how to estimate the log-linear models presented in the previous chapters. In addition, the exploratory analysis of rater agreement is illustrated, and sample LISREL command files are given for the analysis of correlation matrices from different groups of raters. Practically all of the general purpose statistical software packages have modules that allow one to estimate Cohen's κ. Most of these packages also have log-linear modeling modules that are flexible enough to accommodate model specifications as needed for the standard and non-standard log-linear models discussed in this book. In the following sections, we present sample code and sample output for most of the examples given in the first four chapters of this book.

We focus on the six programs SYSTAT 10 (Wilkinson, 2000); SPSS 11 (SPSS, 2001); SAS 8 (SAS, 1999); Lem (Vermunt, 1997); PAW95 (von Eye, 1997); CFA 2000 (von Eye, 2001); and LISREL (Jöreskog & Sörbom, 1993). SYSTAT, SAS, and SPSS are general purpose statistical software packages. Lem is a very general program for the analysis of categorical data. The program allows one to fit both manifest and latent variable models. PAF95 is a program that was originally written for Prediction Analysis (PA; Hildebrand, Laing, & Rosenthal, 1977a; von Eye & Niedermeier, 1999). However, it can be used for the analysis of rater agreement in two-dimensional tables as well. CFA2000 is a program specialized in Configural Frequency Analysis. LISREL is a program for structural equation modeling (SEM; for a comparison with other SEM programs see von Eye & Fuller, 2003).

SYSTAT, SPSS, SAS, and LISREL are commercially available. For SYSTAT, go to http://systat.com/. For SPSS, go to http://www.spss.com. For SAS, go to http://www.sas.com. For LISREL, go to http://www.ssicentral.com/product.htm. Lem can be downloaded free from http://www.kub.nl/faculteiten/fsw/organisatie/departementen/mto/softwa re2.html.

Once at this site, you can download the Lem program, the Lem manual, and examples. The programs PAF95 and CFA2000 can be requested from VONEYE@MSU.EDU. The programs and the CFA manual are free.

The following three sections illustrate the use of SPSS, SYSTAT, and SAS for calculating κ. The log-linear models are then illustrated using Lem. The exploratory analysis of agreement data is illustrated using CFA2000, and the comparison of correlation matrices is demonstrated using LISREL.

5.1   Using SPSS to Calculate Cohen's κ

SPSS is a general purpose statistical software package. It can be used to perform a large number of statistical analyses and to create graphical representations. For the analysis of categorical data, it contains such modules as CROSSTABS and LOGLINEAR. In this section, we illustrate the use of CROSSTABS.

The SPSS module CROSSTABS allows one to analyze quadratic and rectangular two-dimensional tables. A number of statistical coefficients can be calculated, including, for example, X^2, the contingency coefficient, Φ and λ for nominal level data, γ and Somer's d for ordinal level data, and Cohen's κ. For the following illustration, we assume that a frequency table already exists. (If this is not the case, it can be created using SPSS from raw data.)

To input an existing I x J-frequency table, we need to create three variables. The first indicates the rows, the second indicates the columns, and the third indicates the frequencies. Creating variables is easily performed in SPSS's *Variable View* and is not elaborated here. Using the severity-of-depression data from Table 1.2, the following data set is created in *Data View*:

```
1.00     1.00     11.00
1.00     2.00      2.00
```

```
1.00      3.00     19.00
2.00      1.00      1.00
2.00      2.00      3.00
2.00      3.00      3.00
3.00      1.00       .00
3.00      2.00      8.00
3.00      3.00     82.00
```

The first column in this array is the row variable, which indicates the three rating categories used by the first psychiatrist. Because these ratings are crossed with the same ratings of the second psychiatrist, each of the three rating categories appears three times, once for each of the categories used by the second psychiatrist. The rating categories used by the second psychiatrist appear in the second column. The observed frequencies appear in the third column. In the following illustration, we call the first psychiatrist *psy1*, the second psychiatrist *psy2*, and the frequency variable *freq*.

We now need to tell the program how to interpret these data. Specifically, the program needs to be told which of these three variables is the frequency variable. To accomplish this, we click on *Data* and *Weight Cases*. Then we click on *Weight cases by*, the frequency variable *freq*, and the triangle that moves the variable into the little variable window. We then click *OK*, and the program knows that *freq* is the frequency variable.

To estimate κ, we click *Analyze, Descriptive Statistics*, and *Crosstabs*. Within *Crosstabs*, we indicate that *psy1* is the row variable, and that *psy2* is the column variable. Currently, we are only interested in Cohen's kappa. Therefore, we click the *Statistics* button, then check *Cohen's* κ, and *Continue*. The statistics selection window then closes and the results appear on the screen. The following two panels display a slightly edited selection of the output.

The first panel contains the frequency table. The frequencies are the same as in Table 1.2. The zero is not printed. The second panel presents the estimates for κ, its standard error, the *t*-statistic, and the one-sided tail probability. The κ-estimate and its standard error are the same as reported Section 1.2. The file *COMPUTERILLUSTRATIONS 1* on the CD that comes with this text illustrates these steps graphically.

PSY1 * PSY2 Crosstabulation
Count

		PSY2			Total
		1.00	2.00	3.00	
PSY1	1.00	11	2	19	32
	2.00	1	3	3	7
	3.00		8	82	90
Total		12	13	104	129

Symmetric Measures

		Value	Asymp. Std. Error	Approx. T	Approx. Sig.
Measure of Agreement	Kappa	.375	.079	5.943	.000
N of Valid Cases		129			

5.2   Using SYSTAT to Calculate Cohen's κ

SYSTAT is a general purpose statistical software package. We now describe the steps needed to estimate κ.

First, we need to input the data matrix. This can be done in the same way as in SPSS, only labeling the variables is a little different. SYSTAT does not provide the *Variable View* option. Instead, one defines variable names and variable characteristics by clicking *Data* and *Variable Characteristics*. If the data matrix exists in, for example, ASCII or SPSS code, SYSTAT can read these matrices, including the variable names.

We now need to tell SYSTAT, which of the variables is the frequency variable. We click *Data*, *Frequency*, highlight *freq*, and *add* it into the variable window. Clicking *OK* completes the specification of the frequency variable. Clicking *Statistics*, *Crosstabs*, and *Two-way* opens the window for the specification of the cross-classification. We declare *psy1* to be the row variable and *psy2* the column variable. From the *statistics* options, we only select Cohen's κ. We click *Continue* and *OK*, and the results can be had by invoking the *Untitled* button in the selection at the bottom of the screen. The slightly edited output appears in the following two panels.

The top panel of the SYSTAT output reproduces the frequency table. The bottom panel contains first the LR-X^2-statistic and its significance test. For the κ-statistic, only the estimate and its standard error are reported. The z-statistic can be estimated by dividing the coefficient by its standard error. We obtain the same results as in Section 1.2.

```
Frequencies
PSY1 (rows) by PSY2 (columns)
```

	1	2	3	Total
1	11	2	19	32
2	1	3	3	7
3	0	8	82	90
Total	12	13	104	129

```
WARNING: More than one-fifth of fitted cells are sparse (frequency <
5). Significance tests computed on this table are suspect.
```

Test statistic	Value	df	Prob
Pearson Chi-square	42.498	4.000	0.000

Coefficient	Value		Asymptotic Std Error
Cohen Kappa		0.375	0.079

5.3   Programs for Weighted κ

In this section, we illustrate programs for weighted κ. We begin with SAS, one of the more popular general purpose statistical software packages. We illustrate graphically in Section 5.3.1 how κ and weighted κ can be estimated. In Section 5.3.2, we list more programs.

5.3.1   Using SAS to Calculate Cohen's κ and Weighted κ

SAS is a general purpose statistical software package widely used for both exploratory and advanced statistical data analysis. The latest versions of SAS enables more user-friendly and flexible ways of data analysis than before. For the analysis of categorical data, PROC FREQ (also called Table Analysis) and PROC GENMOD can be used. SAS PROC FREQ is equivalent of SPSS CROSSTABS module while SAS PROC GENMOD is roughly equivalent of SPSS LOGLINEAR. Both SPSS LOGLINEAR and SAS GENMOD can be used for multi-way associations among categorical variables. In this section, we illustrate the use of PROC FREQ.

The SAS module PROC FREQ (or Table Analysis) allows one to analyze up to three-way tables with the third variable as stratification variable. Two-dimensional tables or two-dimensional tables conditional on the third variable are analyzed using a number of coefficients, including X^2, measures of association, the Mantel-Haenszel test, and measures of agreement.

Two- or three-dimensional tables can be analyzed using both raw data or frequency data. If raw data are at hand, PROC FREQ or Table Analysis can be used to create frequency tables. With an existing *I* x *J*-frequency table, we create two variables to indicate the row and column variables and one frequency variable. These variables can be created either by directly entering numbers in a data matrix window or importing a spreadsheet to SAS. To enable a new data matrix, click *Solutions*, *Analysis*, and *Analyst*. Then in the new data matrix window, simply plug in numbers as done in SPSS or SYSTAT, and name variables by highlighting the top row and typing in the variable names as desired in place of A, B, and C.

Using the same variable names used for SPSS and SYSTAT, the first column is the row variable, PSY1, the second column is the column variable, PSY2, and the last variable indicates frequency counts. To calculate coefficients of Cohen's κ and weighted κ, click *Statistics*, *Table Analysis*, and highlight and move each of row and column variables to *Row* and *Column*, and then identify the frequency variable as *Cell Count*. And then click *Statistics* option and check *Measures of Agreement*. The sequence of point and click executions is coded as follows:

```
PROC FREQ DATA=RATER.TABLE1 ORDER=INTERNAL;
  TABLES PSY1*PSY2 / AGREE NOPERCENT NOROW;
  WEIGHT FREQ;
RUN;
```

PROC FREQ indicates what we intend to do. *DATA = RATER.TABLE1* indicates that the saved SAS data file exists in a SAS library called RATER and the file name is TABLE1. The next two lines indicate two variables PSY1 and PSY2 are cross-tabulated and the cross-tabulated cells are weighted by a variable called FREQ. The following output presents the edited results of the run.

```
Statistics for Table of psy1 by psy2

Kappa Statistics

Statistic           Value        ASE      95% Confidence Limits
-------------------------------------------------------------------
Simple Kappa        0.3745      0.0789        0.2199        0.5291
Weighted Kappa      0.4018      0.0830        0.2392        0.5644

Sample Size = 129
```

Simple Kappa and Weighted Kappa indicated non-weighted Cohen's κ and weighted κ, respectively. Neither SPSS nor SYSTAT provide an option to calculate weighted kappa at the click of the mouse. SAS provides weighted κ using the following weight formula (Cicchetti & Allison, 1971):

$$w_{ij} = 1 - \frac{\left| C_i - C_j \right|}{C_C - C_1},$$

where C_i and C_j are the category values of the ith row and jth column and C is the number of categories. Weights can be assigned as, for instance, in Table 1.3. Cells with perfect rater agreement are assigned a 1. The adjacent cells, these are the one with small discrepancies, are assigned a 0.5. Cells with larger discrepancies than 1 rating point are assigned a 0.

A graphical illustration of SAS' options for Cohen's κ and $κ_w$ is given in the file *COMPUTERILLUSTRATIONS 1* in the companion CD.

5.3.2   Other Programs for Weighted κ

There exists a number of programs that can be used to calculate weighted κ. Examples include *analyse-it*, a macro integrated in Excel that can be downloaded for free inspection for 30 days from http://www.analyse-it.com/weighted-kappa-test_y.htm .
Free programs for weighted κ can be downloaded, for instance, from http://www.myatt.demon.co.uk/ .

A program that can also be had for free (request from VONEYE@MSU.EDU) is PAF95 (short for Prediction Analysis for Windows 95; von Eye, 1997). This program was originally written for Prediction Analysis (PA). However, because of the similarities between the ∇-statistic (∇ is pronounced 'Del') and its variants used in PA one the one hand, and κ and $κ_w$ on the other, this program can be used to estimate $κ_w$. The following paragraphs explain the relationship between PA's ∇ and $κ_w$.

PA uses I x J-tables to assess the success of predicting one configuration of variable categories from another. Consider the tables that results from crossing the variables A and B. Using this table, PA assesses the success of making predictions from categories of A to categories of B. for example, consider the prediction $a_1 \rightarrow b_2$. Cell $a_1 b_2$ contains those cases that confirm this prediction, and Cells $a_1 b_{\neg 2}$ contains those cases that disconfirm it, where the symbol ¬2 indicates that all cell indices other than 2 are included. A cell with prediction confirming cases is called a *hit cell*. A cell with prediction disconfirming cases is called *error cell*.

The success of this prediction can be assessed by comparing the number of cases that confirm the prediction with the number of cases that had been expected to do so. Measures that capture this aspect of success have been called *proportionate increase in hits* measures (PIH; von Eye & Brandtstädter, 1988a). Alternatively, one can compare the number of disconfirming cases with the expected number of disconfirming cases. Measures that accomplish that have been termed *proportionate reduction in error* measures (PRE; Fleiss, 1981). In the present context, PIH and PRE measures are equivalent.

Proceeding as in Section 1.2, we can define parameter ω_{ij} as

$$\omega_{ij} = \begin{cases} 0 & \text{if } a_i b_j \text{ is a hit cell} \\ 1 & \text{if } a_i b_j \text{ is an error cell} \end{cases}$$

and we obtain a proportionate reduction in error measure, PRE, by

$$PRE = \frac{\theta_1^* - \theta_2^*}{\theta_2^*} = 1 - \frac{\theta_1}{\theta_2},$$

where θ_1 and θ_2 are defined as in Section 1.2 (note that the denominator for this PRE-measure is defined in a way different than for κ). Now, defining

$$\theta_1' = \sum_{ij} (1 - \omega_{ij}) m_{ij},$$

where m_{ij} indicates the frequency in Cell ij, and

$$\theta_2' = \sum_{ij} (1 - \omega_{ij}) \hat{m}_{ij},$$

where $\hat{m}_{ij}$ indicates the estimated expected frequency in Cell ij, one can create a proportionate increase in hits measure, PIH, by

$$PIH = \frac{\theta_1' - \theta_2'}{N - \theta_2'},$$

where N is the sample size.

It can be shown that κ is identical to PRE as defined above. In addition, κ_w is equivalent to PIH even if the weights assume values between 0 and 1. κ is a PRE measure with hit cells located only in the main diagonal. PRE and PIH are more general than κ because the hit cells are not constrained to lie in the main diagonal. In addition, PIH is more general than both κ and PRE because there is no requirement that each row of the two-dimensional matrix must contain a hit cell (von Eye & Brandtstädter, 1988a,b). If each diagonal cell is a hit cell and there are no other hit cells, then κ = PRE = PIH.

To illustrate the use of the program PAF95, we re-analyze the data from Section 1.2. The following commands must be issued to key in the frequency table and to calculate $κ_w$.

Command	Effect
double click shortcut to program PAF95	starts program, opens program window on screen. The program asks for a name for the current run. We type
KAPPAW	and hit ← (the ENTER key). The program then asks for the name of an output file. We type
kappaw.out←	The program then asks whether the data are input interactively or via a file. We will key in the data and type
1←	The program now prompts the number of predictor configurations (= number of categories of the row variable of the agreement table). We type
3←	and the number of criterion configurations (= number of categories of the column variable of the agreement table). We type
3←	The program responds by requesting the observed cell frequencies. We type the frequencies row-wise, each frequency followed by ←
11 ← 2← ... 82←	The program then proposes to save the data for further use. We type
1←	to indicate that we'd like to save the data. On program prompt, we type the file name

kappaw.dat↵	The program responds by presenting the frequency table on the screen and offering the opportunity to correct mis-typed data. For once, we typed correctly, and indicate by typing
2↵	that we don't need to correct the data. The program then presents the estimated expected cell frequencies and asks whether the hit cell pattern, that is, the ω_{ij}-values are input via keyboard or file. We indicate that we will use the keyboard and type
1↵	Upon program prompt, we type the ω_{ij}-values from Table 1.3, row-wise, each frequency followed by ↵
1↵ .5↵ ... .5↵ 1↵	The program then offers to save the hit cell pattern. We type
1	to indicate that we would like to save the scores and indicate the file name by typing
kappaw.hit	and ↵. The program then presents a selection of Prediction Analysis-specific results on the screen and by offering further options. We take none of these options, that is we type four time the sequence
2↵	The program window then closes and we open the result file kappaw.out. This file is written in ASCII and can be opened with any word processor, for example, Notepad or WordPerfect.

What follows is the selection of those results in the output file that are relevant for the current purpose of providing an estimate for κ_w. Those parts of the output file that are not of relevance here, have been edited out.

```
           PREDICTION ANALYSIS OF CROSS-CLASSIFICATIONS
             FORTAN90 program; author: Alexander von Eye

        KAPPAW
        number of predictor levels, p =    3
        number of criterion levels, k =    3
        N =   129.

                        Observed Cell Frequencies
                        -------- ---- -----------
```

```
11.      2.     19.     32.
 1.      3.      3.      7.
 0.      8.     82.     90.
12.     13.    104.    129.
```

                              Expected Frequencies
                              -------- -----------
```
2.98    3.22   25.80
 .65     .71    5.64
8.37    9.07   72.56
```

                    Matrix of Hit and Error Cells
                    ------ -- --- --- ----- -----
```
1.00    .50    .00
 .50   1.00    .50
 .00    .50   1.00
```
                              Descriptive Measures
                              ----------- --------
```
                         PIH1 =       .2042
                         PIH2 =       .4018
                          Del =       .4440
                    Precision =       .2649
                        Scope =      1.0000
```

                         Overall Significance Test
                         ------- ------------ ----
```
                 Test statistic z =      3.2533
           Tail probability for z =       .0006
```

Chi-square tests for model [Predictors][Criteria]
---------- ----- --- ----- ----------------------
```
                 Pearson Chi-square =    42.4976
                        df =   4.       p =   .00000
           Likelihood ratio Chi-square =  39.0276
                        df =   4.       p =   .00000
```

                              CARPE DIEM

Read from the top to the bottom of this print out, we see that the program first identifies itself and prints the name of the run. We then find a protocol of the number of row and column categories, the observed and the expected cell frequencies, and the ω_{ij}-values (in the matrix of hit and error cells). Of the descriptive measures that appear in the following block of results, we are interested in PIH2. This is the PIH measure introduced above. We find the score of PIH = 0.4018. We conclude that the two Psychiatrists agree to over 40% better than expected based on the weighted chance model used to estimate the expected cell frequencies. The z-test in the panel below the descriptive statistics indicates that this increase in hits is significant. The X^2-tests in the last printed panel indicate that the null hypothesis of no association between the two raters must be rejected.

A graphical illustration of the use of the PA program to estimate κ is given in the file *COMPUTERILLUSTRATIONS 1* on the companion CD.

5.4 Using Lem to Model Rater Agreement

The following sections illustrate the use of the program Lem for modeling rater agreement. Lem is a general purpose package for the analysis of nominal, ordinal, or interval level categorical data. The program was written in a DOS environment. However, it runs well under practically all versions of Windows, including W98, Me, NT4.0, W2000, and XP.

For the following examples, we use the log-linear module for manifest variables. More specifically, we cast our rater agreement models in terms of non-hierarchical log-linear models of the form

$$\log m_{ij} = \sum_k \beta_k x_k' ,$$

where m_{ij} is the model frequency in Cell ij, β_k is the parameter for the kth column of the design matrix and x_k' is the kth vector of the design matrix X. Each of the models discussed in this book can be cast in this form. All the λ-, δ-, and β-parameters discussed in this text can be subsumed under the β-parameter of the above equation.

For hierarchical log-linear models, Lem needs at least the following four sets of information:

(1)   number of variables,
(2)   number of categories of each variable,
(3)   model to be estimated, and
(4)   frequency table.

For non-standard log-linear models, the design matrix needs to be specified in addition. There are several options to do this. We use the *des* specification which allows us to input a design matrix in practically the same form as throughout this text. Furthermore, covariates can be specified. In the following sections, we present command files and output files for many of the models discussed in this book, beginning with Section 2.2.

5.4.1 Specifying the Equal Weight and the Weight-by-Response-Category Agreement Models

Lem's response to double-clicking the Lem icon is the presentation of three window frames, the Input frame, the Log frame, and the Output frame. The Input frame is used to key in commands. The Log frame provide a protocol of the computational an iteration process. The Output frame contains the output for completed runs. We select the input frame, in which we type commands. For the *Equal Weight Agreement Model*, we type

```
* equal weight agreement model specified with design matrix
* data: two teachers (Table 2.1)
* A = Teacher A
* B = Teacher B
*
* Note: intercept automatically included
*
man 2
dim 4 4
lab A B
mod {A, B, cov (AB,1)}
des [1 0 0 0 0 1 0 0 0 0 1 0 0 0 0 1]     * cov
dat [4 3 1 0 1 5 2 2 1 1 6 2 0 1 5 6]
```

Reading from the top, we first find seven comment lines. Lines that begin with an asterisk are not interpreted as executable command lines. The comment lines in this example provide a description of the run. When estimating more than just one or two models, comment lines are useful mnemonic aids.

The first command line (no asterisk) states man 2. This statement indicates that there are two manifest variables. These are the two raters whose agreement we model. The second statement, dim 4 4, indicates that each of the two manifest variables has four categories. The statement lab A B specifies the names (labels) for the two variables. This is followed by the model statement, mod {A, B, cov (AB,1)}. The first two terms in the curly bracket indicate that the main effects of variables A and B are part of the model. The term cov (AB,1) indicates that a covariate is part of the model specification. Specifically, the parameter AB indicates that the covariate is for the entire table rather than just for one of the variables that span the table. The second parameter, 1, indicates that one effect is included in the form of a covariate. Because one effect is included, the program expects a covariate that has one times as many elements as cells in the cross-classification. In the present example, the cross-classification has 16 cells. Thus, the covariate must have 16 elements, too.

The following lines contain the covariate scores and the frequencies. Alternatively, this information can be read from files. It is important to memorize that Lem organizes matrices such that the variables that change their index first, are listed first, and so on. For the present examples, which contain mostly two-dimensional tables, this implies that data are organized row-wise instead of column-wise. Fortunately, the only implication for the present purposes is that we need to make sure that the order of matrix elements (frequencies) and covariate elements correspond. A comparison of Tables 2.1 and the model equation in Section 2.3.1 with the two command lines above shows that the elements correspond.

When the command file is complete, one starts the model estimation by clicking *File* and *Run*. Lem responds by placing the results in the Output window. This window contains the following, slightly edited information for the present model:

```
LEM: log-linear and event history analysis with missing data.
Developed by Jeroen Vermunt (c), Tilburg University, The Netherlands.
Version 1.0 (September 18, 1997).

*** INPUT ***

  * equal weight agreement model specified with design matrix
  * data: two teachers (Table 2.1)
  * A = Teacher A
  * B = Teacher B
  *
  * Note: intercept automatically included
  *
  man 2
  dim 4 4
  lab A B
  mod {A, B, cov (AB,1)}
  des [1 0 0 0 0 1 0 0 0 0 1 0 0 0 0 1]     * cov
  dat [4 3 1 0 1 5 2 2 1 1 6 2 0 1 5 6]

*** STATISTICS ***

  Number of iterations = 14
  Converge criterion   = 0.0000005130

  X-squared            = 8.1044 (0.4233)
  L-squared            = 10.0804 (0.2594)
  Cressie-Read         = 8.3867 (0.3966)
  Dissimilarity index  = 0.1554
  Degrees of freedom   = 8
  Log-likelihood       = -101.99997
  Number of parameters = 7 (+1)
  Sample size          = 40.0
  BIC(L-squared)       = -19.4307
  AIC(L-squared)       = -5.9196
  BIC(log-likelihood)  = 229.8221
  AIC(log-likelihood)  = 217.9999

  Eigenvalues information matrix
      58.9007     26.5275     15.1302     11.4565      9.3122      6.2557
         4.9925

*** FREQUENCIES ***

  A B      observed  estimated  std. res.
  1 1        4.000      3.040      0.551
  1 2        3.000      1.457      1.278
  1 3        1.000      2.164     -0.791
  1 4        0.000      1.339     -1.157
```

2 1	1.000	0.960	0.041
2 2	5.000	5.291	-0.126
2 3	2.000	2.317	-0.208
2 4	2.000	1.433	0.474
3 1	1.000	0.813	0.208
3 2	1.000	1.321	-0.279
3 3	6.000	6.653	-0.253
3 4	2.000	1.214	0.714
4 1	0.000	1.188	-1.090
4 2	1.000	1.931	-0.670
4 3	5.000	2.867	1.260
4 4	6.000	6.015	-0.006

*** LOG-LINEAR PARAMETERS ***

* TABLE AB [or P(AB)] *

effect	beta	std err	z-value	exp(beta)	Wald	df	prob
main	0.3956			1.4852			
A							
1	-0.0628	0.3172	-0.198	0.9391			
2	0.0053	0.2958	0.018	1.0053			
3	-0.1609	0.3039	-0.530	0.8513			
4	0.2185			1.2442	0.72	3	0.869
B							
1	-0.4421	0.3516	-1.257	0.6427			
2	0.0439	0.2992	0.147	1.0449			
3	0.4392	0.2741	1.602	1.5515			
4	-0.0410			0.9598	3.09	3	0.377
cov(AB)							
1	1.2212	0.3269	3.736	3.3912	13.95	1	0.000

Read from the top of the printout, Lem first identifies itself and then reproduces the input command file. In the *Statistics* block of information, we find the Pearson $X^2 = 8.10$, the LR-$X^2 = 10.08$, and the Cressie-Read $X^2 = 8.39$. Each of these values is followed by its tail probability in parentheses. In this example, each of the three X^2 statistics suggests retaining the model. This is what we did in Section 2.3.1, above.

The next block of information presents the frequency table. We find the cell indices in the two left hand columns, the observed and the expected cell frequencies in the two middle columns, and the standardized residuals in the right hand column. The latter are defined as Pearson X^2-components, that is, as

$$e_{ij} = \sqrt{\frac{(m_{ij} - \hat{m}_{ij})^2}{\hat{m}_{ij}}} ,$$

where m_{ij} and $\hat{m}_{ij}$ are the observed and the expected cell frequencies, respectively. The expected frequencies are the same as in Table 2.2.

The most important parameter of those printed in the last block that is reproduced here (the block with conditional probabilities, which is also part of the default output, was omitted) is the one for the covariate. The covariate contains the information on the weights that are specified for the diagonal cells of the cross-classification. The corresponding parameter is listed last. Its estimate is 1.22, its standard error is 0.33, and its z-score is 3.74 with $p < 0.01$. These are the values reported in Section 2.3.1. We conclude again that the equal weight agreement model allows us to describe the teachers' agreement well.

A graphical illustration of the use of Lem for the estimation of the equal weight agreement model is given in the file *COMPUTERILLUSTRATIONS 1* on the companion CD.

For the *Weight-by-Response-Category* model we only need to change the covariate vector so that it reflects the differential weights. All the rest of the command file can stay intact. We illustrate this model using the same data as for the example in the previous section. The new command file follows:

```
* equal weight agreement model specified with design matrix
* data: two teachers (Table 2.1)
* A = Teacher A
* B = Teacher B
*
* Note: intercept automatically included
*
man 2
dim 4 4
lab A B
mod {A, B, cov (AB,1)}
des [1 0 0 0 0 2 0 0 0 0 3 0 0 0 0 4]      * cov
dat [4 3 1 0 1 5 2 2 1 1 6 2 0 1 5 6]
```

Readers are invited to run this model. Results will show that this model and the equal weight agreement model fit equally well. There is no statistical way to compare the two models, because they are not hierarchically related. Still, the equal weight agreement model is more parsimonious because it does not specify differential weights. Therefore, we retain the equal weight model.

The use of Lem is illustrated graphically in the file *COMPUTERILLUSTRATIONS 1* in the companion CD to this text.

5.4.2   Models with Covariates

In this section, we illustrate models with covariates. First, we model Graham's (1995) model of categorical covariates, and then models for continuous covariates.

5.4.2.1 Models with Categorical Covariates

The following sample command files reproduce the four runs presented in Section 2.3.3.1, in which we compared concreteness ratings across the two gender groups (data from Table 2.7). Result outputs are not given here. Readers are invited to reproduce the results reported in Section 2.3.3.1 on their computers. The first command file implements the main effect base model, that is, Model 1 in Table 2.8.

```
* two groups of raters, same objects
* data: proverbs (Table 2.7)
* Model 1
* labels:
* A = Proverb 2
* B = Gender
* C = Proverb 1
*
* Constant assumed
*
man 3
dim 2 2 2
lab C B A
mod {A,B,C}
dat [20 23 12 6 8 82 6 25]
```

As can be seen from the five command lines needed to specify this model, there are three manifest variables, each of which has two categories. The variables are labeled A, B, and C. In the model statement, we specify that only main effects are estimated. The last command line contains the frequency table.

The next command file reproduces Model 2 in Table 2.8. This model proposes equal weight agreement that is the same across the two gender groups. In addition, this model includes the associations between Gender and the first proposition and Gender and the second proposition, because the rated propositions were the same across the gender groups. (Please note that the frequencies are arranged in the sequence indicated in the command file. This sequence differs from the one indicated in the text, above. Results are the same, that is, do not depend on the sequence of variables.)

```
* two groups of raters, same objects
* data: proverbs (Table 2.7)
* Model 2
* labels:
* A = Proverb 2
* B = Gender
* C = Proverb 1
*
```

```
* Constant assumed
*
man 3
dim 2 2 2
lab C B A
mod {A,B,C,AB,BC,cov(ABC,1)}
des [1 0 1 0 0 1 0 1]
dat [20 23 12 6 8 82 6 25]
```

The hypothesis that agreement is the same in the two groups, is expressed in the des command. The vector that is added to the design matrix states that the weights in the main diagonal are equal (1) for the first gender group, (2) for the second gender group, and (3) across gender groups. This vector is the result of adding the two vectors that could have been specified to express equal weight hypotheses separately for the two gender groups.

The third command file includes the vector for the gender-specific agreement hypothesis. This is Model 3 in Table 2.8.

```
* two groups of raters, same objects
* data: proverbs (Table 2.7)
* Model 3
* labels:
* A = Proverb 2
* B = Gender
* C = Proverb 1
*
* Constant assumed
*
man 3
dim 2 2 2
lab C B A
mod {A,B,C,AB,BC,cov(ABC,2)}
des [1 0 1 0 0 1 0 1
     1 0 0 0 0 1 0 0]
dat [20 23 12 6 8 82 6 25]
```

The fourth command file presented here is that for Model 4 in Table 2.8. This model includes only the triple superscripted term, that is the second covariate in Model 3.

```
* two groups of raters, same objects
* data: proverbs (Table 2.7)
* Model 4
* labels:
* A = Proverb 2
* B = Gender
* C = Proverb 1
*
* Constant assumed
*
man 3
dim 2 2 2
lab C B A
```

```
mod {A,B,C,AB,BC,cov(ABC,1)}
des [1 0 0 0 0 1 0 0]
dat [20 23 12 6 8 82 6 25]
```

5.4.2.2 Models with Continuous Covariates

This section presents the command files for the agreement models with continuous covariates from Section 2.3.3.2. We use the data from Table 2.9 (severity of depression ratings) and present the command file for Model 3 in Table 2.10. This is the equal weight agreement model with the covariate Severity of Paranoia ratings.

```
* agreement with one continuous covariate
* data: severity of depression (Table 2.9)
* Model 3 (Table 2.10)
* labels:
* A = Psychiatrist 1
* B = Psychiatrist 2
*
* Constant assumed
*
man 2
dim 3 3
lab A B
mod {A,B,cov(AB,2)}
des [1 0 0 0 1 0 0 0 1
     17 27 3 16 45 14 1 3 3]
dat [11 2 19 1 3 3 0 8 82]
```

Note that, in this example, we need two covariates, because both the equal weight agreement vector and the Severity of Paranoia ratings are treated as covariates.

5.4.3   Linear-by-Linear Association Models of Rater Agreement

In this section, we present two sample command files. The first represents a linear-by-linear association equal weight agreement model. The second represents a linear-by-linear association differential weight agreement model with one covariate.

The model in the following sample command file fits the linear-by-linear association equal weight agreement model discussed in Section 2.3.4. We use the data from Table 2.11.

```
* agreement with one continuous covariate
* data: severity of depression (Table 2.11)
* Model 3 (Table 2.12)
* labels:
* A = Journalist 1
```

```
* B = Journalist 2
*
* Constant assumed
*
man 2
dim 6 6
lab A B
mod {A,B,ass(A,B,2a),cov(AB,1)}
des [1 0 0 0 0 0 1 0 0 0 0 0 1 0 0 0 0 0 1 0 0 0 0 0 1 0 0 0
0 0 0 1]
dat [5 8 1 2 4 2 3 5 3 5 5 0 1 2 6 11 2 1 0 1 5 4 3 3 0 0 1 2 5 2 0
0 1 2 1 4]
```

The mod line differs from the ones we used before. Here, this line shows that Lem has provisions for a number of association models. For the present example, we use Option 2, that is, linear-by-linear or uniform association, and a, that is, homogeneous interaction. The equal weights in the main diagonal are expressed in the first line of the des specification. The covariate appears in the second line of the des specification; both are in the same pair of brackets. The 2 in the cov parentheses indicates that two covariate vectors are specified. (Please note that the results created using this command file differ from the ones reported in Section 2.3.4, which were created using SPSS. Lem encounters identification problems, SPSS does not (and neither does SAS).

The second model presented in this section is the linear-by-linear association differential weight agreement model with one covariate. We use the data from Table 2.13 and the weights and the covariate listed in the text under Table 2.13 in Section 2.3.5, and we fit Model 4 in Table 2.14.

```
* agreement with one continuous covariate
* data: severity of carcinoma (Table 2.13)
* Model 4 (Table 2.14)
* labels:
* A = Pathologist 1
* B = Pathologist 2
*
* Constant assumed
*
man 2
dim 4 4
lab A B
mod {A,B,ass(A,B,2a),cov(AB,2)}
des [4 0 0 0 0 1 0 0 0 0 1 0 0 0 0 4
      1.4 2 2.2 0 2.1 2.2 2 0 0 2.2 2.5 0 0 2.2 2.3 1.7]
dat [22 2 2 0 5 7 14 0 0 2 36 0 0 1 17 10]
```

5.4.4   Models of Agreement among More than Two Raters

In this section, we present sample command files for models of agreement among three raters. The first command file represents a model in which three raters are simultaneously compared both in pairs and as a triplet. We use the data from Table 3.6 and the most complete of the two comparison models discussed in Sections 2.4.1.1 and 2.4.1.2. The model is cast in terms of a model with four covariates. The first three covariates, given in the first three lines of the des command, model agreement between Psychiatrists 1 and 2, Psychiatrists 1 and 3, and Psychiatrists 2 and 3. The fourth line models the agreement in the triplet of the three raters. The fourth of these lines must be dropped when only agreement in pairs of raters is of interest. The first three lines must be dropped if only agreement in the triplet of raters is of interest (Section 2.4.1.2).

```
* equal weight agreement model for three pairs of raters
* data: psychiatrist's re-diagnoses (Table 3.6)
* three raters, simultaneous pairs
* A = Rater A
* B = Rater B
* C = Rater C
*
* Note: intercept assumed
man 3
dim 3 3 3
lab A B C
mod {A,B,C,cov(ABC,4)}
des [1 1 1 0 0 0 0 0 0 0 0 0 1 1 1 0 0 0 0 0 0 0 0 0 1 1 1
     1 0 0 1 0 0 1 0 0 0 1 0 0 1 0 0 1 0 0 1 0 0 0 1 0 0 1
     1 0 0 0 1 0 0 0 1 1 0 0 0 1 0 0 0 1 1 0 0 0 1 0 0 0 1
     1 0 0 0 0 0 0 0 0 0 0 0 1 0 0 0 0 0 0 0 0 0 0 0 0 0 1]
dat [4 3 6 2 1 3 2 2 17 0 1 2 1 1 1 0 0 4 0 1 3 0 1 8 0 4 96]
```

5.4.5   Models of Rater-Specific Trends

The command file presented in this section represents the rater-specific trend model discussed in Section 2.4.2. we use the data from Table 2.16 and design matrix given in the text above the table. The first of the covariate vectors models the equal weight agreement hypothesis. The second vector models the trend hypothesis.

```
* diagonal set model specified with design matrix
* data: diagnoses
* rater trend agreement model
* A = Rater A
* B = Rater B
*
* Note: intercept assumed
```

```
*
man 2
dim 3 3
lab A B
mod {A,B,cov(AB,2)}
des [1 0 0 0 1 0 0 0 1
     0 1 1 -1 0 1 -1 -1 0]
dat [17 27 3 16 45 14 1 3 3]
```

5.5 Using Configural Frequency Analysis to Explore Patterns of Agreement

The program CFA 2000 (von Eye, 2001) allows one to perform CFA searches for types and antitypes. The program is interactive. It allows one to read in raw data or frequency tables. If needed, variables can be dichotomized at the median or split at user-specified cut-offs. In the present context, we illustrate CFA using four examples. For each of the examples, we assume that a frequency table exists before analysis. The first example uses a log-linear main effect model as a base model. The second example uses a log-linear null model for a base model. the third example includes a covariate. The fourth example analyzes three raters.

5.5.1 First Order CFA (Main Effects Only)

We illustrate the example of an exploratory analysis of rater agreement using the data from Table 3.1. The CFA program is started by double-clicking the program icon in the computer screen. The program opens a window and asks the user questions that must be answered using the key board. The following commands are issued to analyze the data in Table 3.1.

Command	Effect
	After starting the program, it asks whether data will be input via file (=1) or interactively, via the keyboard (=2). We select interactive data input and type
2 ←	The program now asks for the number of variables to be processed. We type

2↵	The program now asks for the number of categories for the first variable. We type
3↵	Prompted, we indicate the number of categories for the second variable by typing
3↵	The program now asks for the individual cell frequencies. We type each frequency, followed by ↵, that is, in the present example,
11↵ 2↵ ... 8↵ 82↵	After all cell frequencies are typed in, the program gives the sample size, in the present example $N = 129$, and asks whether the user wishes to save the data (yes = 1, no = 2). We indicate that we wish to save the data and type
1↵	The program then asks for the name of the file in which we wish to save the data. We type
depress.dat ↵	A total of 80 spaces can be used for the file name. Now, the program presents the currently available CFA base models. All we need for the present example is the main effect model, also called a *first order CFA base model*. We indicate this by typing
1↵	The program now presents the univariate marginal frequencies on the screen. In the present example, these are the frequencies with which each rater used the rating categories. In addition, the program asks whether the user wishes to include a covariate, and indicates the maximum number of covariates that can be included in a particular run. We do not have a covariate and indicate that by typing
2↵	The program follows up by presenting the currently available statistical tests. To replicate the results in Table 3.1, we select the normal approximation of the binomial test. To indicate this choice, we type
5↵	The program then asks for the nominal significance threshold, α. We type

.05↵	At the question concerning the name of the output file, we type
depress.out↵	As for the input file, a total of 80 spaces can be used for the output file name. The program now writes the results to the output file, and then asks whether the user wishes to include the design matrix in the output file. We indicate that yes by typing
1↵	This concludes the CFA run and the program window closes.

The saved data file is reproduced in the following panel:

```
2   3   3
   11.
    2.
   19.
    1.
    3.
    3.
    0.
    8.
   82.
```

The first line in this file contains the number of variables and the number of categories for each variable. The sample run resulted in the following, slightly edited output file, depress.out:

```
                    Configural Frequency Analysis
                    ---------- --------- --------
          author of program: Alexander von Eye, 2002

    Marginal Frequencies
    --------------------
    Variable Frequencies
    -------- -----------
         1      32.    7.    90.
         2      12.   13.   104.

  sample size N =       129
  the normal approximation of the binomial test was used
  Bonferroni-adjusted alpha =   .0055556
  a CFA of order   1  was performed

                            Table of results
                            ----- -- -------
    Configuration      fo       fe   statistic      p
    -------------     ----   -------- ---------   -------
           11         11.     2.977     4.705    .00000127    Type
           12          2.     3.225     -.691    .24486524
```

```
          13          19.    25.798    -1.496    .06726707
          21           1.      .651      .433    .33236650
          22           3.      .705     2.739    .00307695    Type
          23           3.     5.643    -1.138    .12757930
          31           0.     8.372    -2.992    .00138503    Antitype
          32           8.     9.070     -.368    .35628691
          33          82.    72.558     1.676    .04689376

              chi2 for CFA model =    42.4976
              df =       4        p =  .00000001
          LR-chi2 for CFA model =     39.0276
              df =       4        p =  .00000007
```

Descriptive indicators of types and antitypes
----

cell	Rel. Risk	Rank	logP	Rank
11	3.695	2	3.563	1
12	.620	7	.140	9
13	.736	6	.711	5
21	1.536	3	.321	6
22	4.253	1	1.458	3
23	.532	8	.234	8
31	.000	9	1.483	2
32	.882	5	.318	7
33	1.130	4	1.097	4

Design Matrix
------ ------

```
  .0      .0    1.0    1.0
  .0     1.0    1.0     .0
  .0    -1.0    1.0    -1.0
 1.0      .0     .0    1.0
 1.0     1.0     .0     .0
 1.0    -1.0     .0    -1.0
-1.0      .0    -1.0    1.0
-1.0     1.0    -1.0     .0
-1.0    -1.0    -1.0    -1.0
```

                                    CARPE DIEM

Reading from the top to the bottom of the output file, we first find that the program identifies itself, and then presents the marginal frequencies and the sample size we had seen already on the screen. In addition, there is a protocol of the specifications made for the current run. What follows is the results table that was reported in Table 3.1. The left-most column contains the indices for the configurations (= cell indices). The second column, it has the header fo, contains the observed cell frequencies. The third column, it has the header fe, displays the expected cell frequencies which were estimated under the main effect base model. The cell-specific z-statistics appear in the fourth column, followed by their one-sided tail probabilities. In the last column, cells that constitute types and cells that constitute antitypes are marked es such.

Under the table, we find the Pearson- and the likelihood ratio X^2-

statistics, their degrees of freedom, and their tail probabilities. As a rule of thumb, types and antitypes can emerge only if the X^2-statistics indicate significant data-model discrepancies.

The following table displays the Relative Risk and the logP statistics for each cell. Here, we don't need these results and move on the design matrix at the end of the printout. This matrix contains the four column vectors needed for the main effects of the 3 x 3 table under study.

The use of the program CFA2000 is graphically illustrated in the file *COMPUTERILLUSTRATIONS 1* on the companion CD.

5.5.2   Zero Order CFA

The second example uses zero order CFA as a base model. We reproduce the example in Table 3.2, and issue the following commands.

Command	Effect
	After starting the program, it asks whether data will be input via file (=1) or interactively, via the keyboard (=2). We select input via file and type
1 ↵	The program now asks whether a raw data file or a frequency table is being read. We type
2↵	to indicate that we are reading a frequency table. We are reading the table that we saved in the first example, that is file
depress.dat↵	The program responds by presenting a description of the data file, the sample size, and by presenting the options for base models. We type
0↵	to indicate that we are interested in a zero order CFA. The program follows up by offering to include covariates. We type
2↵	to indicate that this run does not include covariates. The program now lists the currently available statistical tests. To replicate the results in Table 3.2, we select the normal approximation of the binomial test. To indicate this choice, we type

5↵	The program then asks for the nominal significance threshold, α. We type
.05↵	At the question concerning the name of the output file, we type
depressz.out ↵	The program now writes the results to the output file, and then asks whether the user wishes to include the design matrix in the output file. We indicate that yes by typing
1↵	This concludes the CFA run and the program window closes.

The following panel contains the slightly edited output file (descriptive indicators of types and antitypes omitted).

```
                  Configural Frequency Analysis
                  ---------- --------- --------
          author of program: Alexander von Eye, 2002

      Marginal Frequencies
      --------------------
      Variable Frequencies
      -------- -----------
         1      32.    7.     90.
         2      12.   13.    104.

    sample size N =      129
   the normal approximation of the binomial test was used
   Bonferroni-adjusted alpha =   .0055556
   a CFA of order   0  was performed


                          Table of results
                          ----- -- -------
   Configuration    fo       fe    statistic      p
   -------------    ---    -------- ---------    -------
         11        11.    14.333     -.934     .17518826
         12         2.    14.333    -3.455     .00027491    Antitype
         13        19.    14.333     1.307     .09553803
         21         1.    14.333    -3.735     .00009372    Antitype
         22         3.    14.333    -3.175     .00074893    Antitype
         23         3.    14.333    -3.175     .00074893    Antitype
         31         0.    14.333    -4.016     .00002966    Antitype
         32         8.    14.333    -1.774     .03800404
         33        82.    14.333    18.957     .00000000    Type


            chi2 for CFA model =   379.8140
              df =     8      p =    .00000000

          LR-chi2 for CFA model =   249.6237
              df =     8      p =    .00000000
```

```
Design Matrix
------ ------
```

Reading from the top to the bottom of the output file, we find the program identification, the marginal frequencies, the sample size, and the specifications made for the current run. The result table follows (see Table 3.2). The columns of this table contain, from left to right, the cell indices, the observed frequencies, the estimated expected frequencies, the z-statistics, their one-sided tail probabilities, and the labeling of those cells that constitute types or antitypes. The estimated expected cell frequencies indicate that the null model that is used in zero order CFA uses only the sample size as information. The expected distribution is therefore uniform. The design matrix at the bottom of the output seems to be empty. It only contains the vector of 1s which is not printed. There are no other vectors in this matrix.

5.5.3   First Order CFA with One Continuous Covariate

The third CFA example uses the same base model as the first (Section 5.5.1). However, it includes a covariate. For the following illustration, we use the data from Section 2.3.3.2 and the covariate that is listed in the paragraph before Table 2.9. We issue the following commands.

Command	Effect
	The program asks whether the data will be input interactively or via a file. In the example in the Section 5.5.1, we saved the data in a file, so we use this file for the present run. We type
1↵	to indicate that data input will be via file. The program asks whether raw data are going to be read or a frequency table. Typing
2↵	we indicate that the data are in the form of a frequency table. The program now needs to know the name of the data file. We type

depress.dat↵	The program responds by indicating the number of categories per variable, and the sample size. It then presents the currently available base models. We select the main effect model by tying
1↵	The program now presents the marginal frequencies and asks whether we wish to include a covariate. The answer is yes and we type
1↵	The program now prompts the scores of the covariate cell-by-cell. We type
17↵27↵ ... 3↵3↵	that is, the scores from the covariate vector in Section 2.3.3.2. The program offers to take into account another covariate. We decline and type
2↵	The program then presents the selection of significance tests. We type
4↵	to indicate that we use the z-test. The program now asks for the significance level. We type
.05↵	To the question concerning the name of the output file we respond by typing
depressc.out ↵	The program's last question is whether we wish to include the design matrix in the output file. We indicate yes by typing
1↵	The program window closes and the output file is ready.

The output file follows, in slightly edited form.

```
              Configural Frequency Analysis
              ---------- --------- --------
        author of program: Alexander von Eye, 2002

    Marginal Frequencies
    --------------------
    Variable Frequencies
    -------- -----------
       1        32.     7.     90.
       2        12.    13.    104.

  sample size N =      129
```

```
the normal z-test was used
Bonferroni-adjusted alpha =   .0055556
a CFA of order   1  was performed

                                Table of results
                                ----- -- -------
Configuration       fo        fe  statistic        p
--------------      ----  --------  ---------     -------
           11       11.     5.411      2.402   .00814406
           12        2.     6.607     -1.792   .03654584
           13       19.    19.982      -.220   .41307503
           21        1.      .440       .845   .19909749
           22        3.     2.390       .394   .34663192
           23        3.     4.170      -.573   .28333168
           31        0.     6.149     -2.480   .00657501
           32        8.     4.003      1.998   .02287402
           33       82.    79.848       .241   .40484921

                 chi2 for CFA model =    20.4272
                 df =       3        p =  .00013842
              LR-chi2 for CFA model =    25.3820
                 df =       3        p =  .00001285

Descriptive indicators of types and antitypes
---------------------------------------------
       cell  Rel. Risk  Rank        logP    Rank
     --------  ---------  ----      ----    ----
           11     2.033     2       1.652       1
           12      .303     8        .464       6
           13      .951     6        .470       5
           21     2.274     1        .449       7
           22     1.255     4        .381       8
           23      .719     7        .183       9
           31      .000     9        .859       3
           32     1.998     3       1.298       2
           33     1.027     5        .797       4

Design Matrix
------ ------
   .0     .0    1.0    1.0   17.0
   .0    1.0    1.0     .0   27.0
   .0   -1.0    1.0   -1.0    3.0
  1.0     .0     .0    1.0   16.0
  1.0    1.0     .0     .0   45.0
  1.0   -1.0     .0   -1.0   14.0
 -1.0     .0   -1.0    1.0    1.0
 -1.0    1.0   -1.0     .0    3.0

 -1.0   -1.0   -1.0   -1.0    3.0

                    CARPE DIEM
```

Reading from the top of the output, we find the program identification, the marginal frequencies, the sample size, and a summary of the specifications for this run. The result table follows. It should be noted that the expected cell frequencies in the present example differ from the ones in Table 2.9. The reason for this difference is that the model in Table 2.9 included the parameter δ for the equal weight agreement hypothesis. The vector that represents this parameter is not part of the CFA base model, because in CFA, beyond-expectation agreement emerges in the form of types that contradict a particular base model. Therefore, hypotheses concerning the main diagonal are typically not modeled. The present analysis reveals no types or antitypes. We thus conclude that there is no agreement that is stronger than chance in any of the diagonal cells. In addition, there is no antitype.

The X^2-tests under the results table indicate significant model-data differences. However, none of the individual differences was big enough to constitute a type or antitype.

The design matrix at the end of the output contains five columns. The first four display the four vectors that are needed for the main effects of the four rating categories. The last column contains the scores for the covariate. Readers are invited to inspect the expected cell frequencies when the vector that represents the linear-by-linear association between the severity ratings is also included. This vector is $x_7' = [1, 2, 3, 2, 4, 6, 3, 6, 9]$.

5.5.4   CFA of the Agreement in Two Groups; No Gender-Association Base Model

In this section, we reproduce the analysis for Table 3.5. We ask whether the agreement patterns concerning two proverbs are the same across the two gender groups. This base model requires that the interactions that include Gender with the first proverb, Gender with the second proverb, and Gender with both proverbs are not part of the parameters that are estimated. Only the Proverb1 x Proverb2 interaction is included. To include this part of the model, the last vector of the design matrix in the paragraphs before Table 3.5 has to be keyed in, in the form of a covariate. As in the CFA base models before, there is no provision for parameters concerning the main diagonals of the agreement matrices. Agreement types will emerge if agreement is beyond chance in any of the diagonal cells. The following commands are issued after starting the CFA program.

Command	Effect
	The program first asks whether the data will be put in via a file or interactively. We indicate that we will type the data in and type

2↵   The programs asks for the number of variables. We
                     type

3↵   The program next needs to know the number of
                     categories of each variable. We respond to the first
                     prompt by typing

2↵   This is repeated three times, until all three variables
                     are covered. Next, the program asks for the cell
                     frequencies. We type

20↵23↵ ...   The program now asks whether we wish to save the
6↵25↵   data. We indicate that yes by typing

1↵   At the prompt, we indicate that

provgen.dat   is the name of the data file. The program next asks
                     what level CFA base model we wish to use. We
                     indicate that we will run a first order model, that is, a
                     main effect only model (the two interactions are
                     included as covariates), by typing

1↵   The program then asks whether we wish to include a
                     covariate. The answer is yes and we type

1↵   At the prompt, we then type the covariate scores from
                     the last column of the design matrix in Section 3.2.3,

1↵-1↵-1↵ ...   The program offers the option of a second covariate.
-1↵-1↵1↵   We accept and type

2↵   to indicate that we do not use a second covariate.
                     From the displayed significance tests, we select the z-
                     test and type

4↵   We then indicate that the nominal significance level
                     is

.05↵   The name of the output file is

provgen.out   Finally, to obtain the design matrix in the output file,
↵   we type

1↵	The window closes and we look at the output file.

What follows is the slightly edited output file of the above example (descriptors of types and antitypes omitted).

```
                    Configural Frequency Analysis
                    ---------- --------- --------
          author of program: Alexander von Eye, 2002

     Marginal Frequencies
     --------------------
     Variable Frequencies
     -------- -----------
         1      133.     49.
         2       61.    121.
         3       46.    136.

   sample size N =        182
 Pearsons chi2 test was used
  Bonferroni-adjusted alpha =   .0062500
  a CFA of order   1  was performed

                                   Table of results
                                   ----- -- -------
     Configuration     fo       fe   statistic      p
     -------------     ----    --------- ---------  -------
         111          20.     23.385      .490    .48398152
         112          23.     21.192      .154    .69455813
         121           8.     10.231      .486    .48553389
         122          82.     78.192      .185    .66675507
         211          12.      8.615     1.330    .24886393
         212           6.      7.808      .419    .51767161
         221           6.      3.769     1.320    .25054703
         222          25.     28.808      .503    .47805967


                 chi2 for CFA model =    4.8876
                 df =      3      p =   .18021203

               LR-chi2 for CFA model =    4.6568
                 df =      3      p =   .19872596

Design Matrix
------ ------
   1.0    1.0    1.0    1.0
   1.0    1.0   -1.0   -1.0
   1.0   -1.0    1.0   -1.0
   1.0   -1.0   -1.0    1.0
  -1.0    1.0    1.0    1.0
  -1.0    1.0   -1.0   -1.0
  -1.0   -1.0    1.0   -1.0
  -1.0   -1.0   -1.0    1.0
                        CARPE DIEM
```

The table with the main results reproduces Table 3.5 exactly. It indicates that not a single gender-specific pattern of agreement exists. The last column of the design matrix contains the Proverb1 x Proverb2 interaction taken into account.

5.5.5   CFA of the Agreement among Three Raters

Using CFA for the exploratory analysis of the agreement among three raters goes along the lines described in the previous sections. Here, we only list the commands issued to perform the analysis of the data in Table 3.8. For results see Table 3.8. When three raters are compared, we cross their ratings and obtain an I x I x I-table. The base model is that of rater independence. The commands for CFA follow.

Command	Effect
	We indicate that we will key in the frequency table by typing
1↵	We indicate the number of variables by typing
3↵	Each of the variables in the present example has three categories. We type
3↵	and repeat this procedure twice. To enter the frequencies from Table 3.8, we type
4↵3↵6↵ ... 4↵96↵	Once the data are completely entered, we indicate that we would like to save them by typing
1↵	We give the data file the name
threerate.dat ↵	and select the first order CFA base model by typing
1↵	In this run there are no covariates. Therefore, we type
2↵	Because of the small sample size, we select the binomial test and type
1↵	and the nominal significance threshold is
.05↵	We give the name for the output file as

threerate.out	and request the design matrix in the output file by
←	typing

1←	This concludes the specifications for this run. The window closes and we can look at the results in the output file.

The output file threerate.out follows, in slightly edited form (descriptive information and design matrix omitted):

```
              Configural Frequency Analysis
              ---------- --------- --------
        author of program: Alexander von Eye, 2002


     Marginal Frequencies
     --------------------
     Variable Frequencies
     -------- -----------
         1      40.    10.    113.
         2      20.    18.    125.
         3       9.    14.    140.

  sample size N =       163
  Bonferroni-adjusted alpha =  .0018519
  a CFA of order   1   was performed
  significance testing used   binomial test


                             Table of results
                             ----- -- -------
  Configuration      fo      fe         p
  -------------      ----    --------   ---------
       111           4.      .271       .00017540     Type
       112           3.      .422       .00901272
       113           6.     4.215       .24767745
       121           2.      .244       .02521266
       122           1.      .379       .31602350
       123           3.     3.794       .47281845
       131           2.     1.694       .50592450
       132           2.     2.635       .50847878
       133          17.    26.346       .02518336
       211           0.      .068       .93448266
       212           1.      .105       .10005359
       213           2.     1.054       .28410874
       221           1.      .061       .05916239
       222           1.      .095       .09051337
       223           1.      .948       .61373980
       231           0.      .423       .65443912
       232           0.      .659       .51685302
       233           4.     6.587       .20839681
       311           0.      .766       .46423831
       312           1.     1.191       .66568033
       313           3.    11.909       .00188667
       321           0.      .689       .50134602
       322           1.     1.072       .70929029
```

```
       323          8.     10.718        .24916846
       331          0.      4.785        .00777889
       332          4.      7.443        .13031872
       333         96.     74.429        .00047052        Type
```

```
              chi2 for CFA model =      140.3746
              df =      20         p =   .00000000
              LR-chi2 for CFA model =    75.1015
              df =      20         p =   .00000003
```

                         CARPE DIEM

5.6   Correlation Structures: LISREL Analyses

LISREL is a program that requires command file input. The following
panel contains the command file that was used to compare the correlation
matrices that had been provided by the girls and boys in the Ohannessian
et al. (1995) study.

```
Testing equality of correlational structures
Rater: girls
DA ng=2 ni=9 no=74
la
FAA FAM FAF FCA FCM FCF FADA FADM FADF
km
1
.30 1
.20 .41 1
.63 .14 .21 1
.38 .72 .29 .07 1
.03 .40 .60 .19 .52 1
.40 .02 -.03 .56 .02 .06 1
.40 .26 .14 .27 .55 .25 .25 1
.35 .03 .11 .32 .08 .13 .37 .52 1
mo nx=9 ph=st,fr
ou rs mi me=ml it=100
Testing equality of correlational structures
Rater: boys
da no= 74
la
FAA FAM FAF FCA FCM FCF FADA FADM FADF
km
1
.26 1
.07 .32 1
.58 .24 .09 1
.03 .35 .12 .26 1
-.05 .17 .51 .21 .33 1
.29 .06 .03 .60 .29 .05 1
-.31 .13 .12 -.09 .22 .2 .09 1
-.02 .02 .49 .01 .33 .36 .12 .49 1
mo ph=in td=sy,fi
fr td 1 1 td 2 2 td 3 3 td 4 4 td 5 5 td 6 6 td 7 7 td 8 8 td 9 9
fr td 5 1 td 8 1 td 9 5 td 9 3
ou mi rs me=ml it=100
```

In the following paragraphs, we explain the LISREL command file for the example in Chapter 5. The comments focus on the example. For more detail and more program options, see Jöreskog and Sörbom (1993).

Reading from the top to the bottom of the LISREL command file, the first line is the *TITLE line*. This line is optional and is not interpreted as a command for LISREL to execute. If one tests more than one model, this line is useful as a mnemonic aid. The second line is a comment line also, useful in multigroup analyses to label the groups. Here, we indicate that the first group whose data are read is the group of the girls. The third line is the *DATA line*. DA is short for DATA. NG is short for "number of groups." Here, we analyze two groups. NI is short for "number of indicators." This is the total number of variables in the input. This number is not necessarily the same as the number used in a model, because later in the command file, one can select variables (an option not used in this example). NO is short for "number of observations." Here, we analyze the responses given by 74 girls. The following line is the *LABEL line*. Specifying LA indicates that labels for the indicators follow, beginning with the next line. For each label, eight spaces can be used. Separation of labels is done by spaces or commas. In the next line, we indicate by "KM" that the input matrix is a correlation matrix. Other options include covariance matrices or raw data matrices. Only the lower triangular of symmetric matrices needs to be given, including the 1s in the diagonal.

The first line after the correlation matrix is the *MODEL line*, abbreviated by MO. NX is the number of variables on the x-side of the model. the LISREL model allows one to distinguish between the x- and the y-sides of a model. The x-side contains the independent variables. The y-side contains the mediators and the dependent variables. The example discussed here requires only one side of the model. It can be specified as a model on the x-side, but could have been specified equivalently on the y-side. PH is short for Φ (Phi). This is the matrix of correlations among the variables under study. Here, we specify Phi to be *st*, that is, a standard correlation matrix with 1s in the diagonal and correlation coefficients on the off-diagonal cells, and *fr*, that is, free. When a matrix is specified as free, all its entries will be estimated.

The following line is the *OUTPUT line* (OU). In this example, we request, the residuals (rs), modification indices (mi), and we tell the program to stop if more than 100 iterations are needed for parameter estimation. This concludes the model specification for the girls' sample.

The second command block in this file contains the specifications for the boys' sample. In LISREL's multisample module, commands and specifications that are identical across groups do not need to be repeated. In the data line, we read that there are 74 boys in the sample. The variable labels are the same as before (omitting the labels encourages the program to use its own labels which, in a multigroup analysis, can be confusing). After the correlation matrix, we find the Model line. PH = in indicates that we want the program to estimate the correlation matrix to be identical across the two groups. This part of the model specification contains the formulation of the null hypothesis that the girls and the boys from the families that participated in the study by Ohannessian et al. (1995) have identical views of the functioning of their families, as indicated by the correlation structures of their responses.

This is a strong hypothesis, bound to be rejected. Indeed, the fit of the model that specified all parameters to be exactly the same was poor. Therefore, we considered the following modification option. We specified the matrix Θ_δ, the residual variance-covariance matrix on the x-side, to be symmetric (sy) and fixed (fi). This matrix is naturally symmetric, as are all covariance matrices. We declare it fixed, just to be able to free entries as needed. In the next line, we free all diagonal elements, thus indicating that portions of the variables variances are left unexplained. In the girls sample, the Θ_δ matrix was not mentioned, because its diagonal is free and its off-diagonal cells are zero by default.

Thus far, the two samples still do not differ. The following line in the command file, however, specifies off-diagonal elements in the boys' Θ_δ-matrix to be freed. These elements are zero in the girls sample. Four elements are set free. The modification indices provided in the earlier runs served as guides. In the present model, there are no large modification indices left. Therefore, and because of the good overall fit indices, we retain the present solution. The output file is too long to be reproduced here entirely. However, we reproduce the parts that provide information about overall model fit. We begin with the overall goodness-of-fit information for the girls. The following, slightly edited panel is taken from the LISREL output file.

```
Testing equality of correlational structures

  Number of Iterations = 20
  LISREL Estimates (Maximum Likelihood)
  PHI EQUALS PHI IN THE FOLLOWING GROUP

              Group Goodness of Fit Statistics

            Contribution to Chi-Square = 17.36
      Percentage Contribution to Chi-Square = 45.04
        Root Mean Square Residual (RMR) = 0.10
```

```
                    Standardized RMR = 0.11
            Goodness of Fit Index (GFI) = 0.95
```

The output indicates that maximum likelihood (ML) was used to estimated the parameters. ML is the default option. The output also indicates that the two Phi matrices are specified to be equal. The girls part of the model contributes 17.36 X^2-units to the overall X^2. This is 45.05 %. The GFI is 0.95, well above the threshold of 0.90 that must be surpassed for a model to be retainable. The corresponding output for the boys sample follows.

```
              Group Goodness of Fit Statistics

              Contribution to Chi-Square = 21.19
        Percentage Contribution to Chi-Square = 54.96

         Root Mean Square Residual (RMR) = 0.091
                   Standardized RMR = 0.083
            Goodness of Fit Index (GFI) = 0.94
```

The contribution of the boys sample to the overall goodness-of-fit X^2 is somewhat larger than for the girls. This indicates that the model of identical correlation matrices describes the girls sample a little better than the boys sample. Still, the GFI for the boys data is 0.94, a value that can be interpreted as in support of the model. The next, slightly edited panel displays the global goodness of fit statistics, that is, the fit information for the model as a whole.

```
              Global Goodness of Fit Statistics

                  Degrees of Freedom = 32
         Minimum Fit Function Chi-Square = 38.55 (P = 0.20)
  Normal Theory Weighted Least Squares Chi-Square = 36.77 (P = 0.26)
          Estimated Non-centrality Parameter (NCP) = 4.77
        90 Percent Confidence Interval for NCP = (0.0 ; 23.99)

                Minimum Fit Function Value = 0.26
          Population Discrepancy Function Value (F0) = 0.035
          90 Percent Confidence Interval for F0 = (0.0 ; 0.18)
      Root Mean Square Error of Approximation (RMSEA) = 0.047
      90 Percent Confidence Interval for RMSEA = (0.0 ; 0.10)
        P-Value for Test of Close Fit (RMSEA < 0.05) = 0.63

           Expected Cross-Validation Index (ECVI) = 1.12
       90 Percent Confidence Interval for ECVI = (1.08 ; 1.26)
                 ECVI for Saturated Model = 0.66
               ECVI for Independence Model = 3.84

  Chi-Square for Independence Model with 72 Degrees of Freedom = 508.15
                    Independence AIC = 544.15
                        Model AIC = 152.77
                      Saturated AIC = 180.00
                    Independence CAIC = 616.10
```

```
Model CAIC = 384.61
Saturated CAIC = 539.75

Normed Fit Index (NFI) = 0.92
Non-Normed Fit Index (NNFI) = 0.97
Parsimony Normed Fit Index (PNFI) = 0.41
Comparative Fit Index (CFI) = 0.98
Incremental Fit Index (IFI) = 0.99
Relative Fit Index (RFI) = 0.83

Critical N (CN) = 203.60
```

Practically all of the overall goodness-of-fit results support the model. Specifically, neither X^2 suggests significant model-data discrepancies. The root mean squared error of approximation (RMSEA) is smaller than 0.05, thus suggesting close fit ($p = 0.63$). The fit indices are all in the desired brackets. We thus retain the model of equal correlation matrices with the proviso that four of the residual correlations had to be free in the boys sample. The reasons for this deviation need to be investigated in a different context.

A graphical illustration of the use of LISREL for the comparison of two correlation matrices is given in the file *COMPUTERILLUSTRATIONS 1* on the companion CD.

5.7 Calculating the Intraclass Correlation Coefficient

The Intraclass correlation coefficient is provided as a standard feature in the SPSS and the SYSTAT software package. In SYSTAT, the ICC is part of the mixed regression module, that is, the module that estimates hierarchical linear regression models (see Section 4.1 of this book). No other software package mentioned in this book includes ICC as a standard feature, although there are a few macros developed for SAS users. The following examples use SPSS.

The data to be analyzed should be arranged in the SPSS data editor like the ones in Table 4.1. And then click *Analyze, Scale,* and *Reliability Analysis.* Highlight the variables that indicate raters or measures and move them to the right side box, called *Items.* Then click *Statistics.* In the *ANOVA* table, check *F test* to get an ANOVA table. In the bottom left of the active window, check *Intraclass correlation coefficient,* which enables more options. *Model* and *Type* need to be determined by the nature of the data and research question. SPSS specifies *Two-way mixed* and *Consistency* as default options. Two-way random and Two-way fixed models would be the most common choice for ICC. Although both models are defined differently at the population model, the ICCs for both models are estimated using the same computational formula. When absolute agreement ICC is of interest, pull down the menu and select *Absolute Agreement*. The following output results for the data in Tables 4.3 and 4.4. Note that there are one ANOVA table and two measures of ICCs in the output. The ANOVA table is the same across all models and types of ICC. Both ICC estimates are significant and high in magnitude, indicating the rank-orders on the six cases by four different raters were pretty consistent. If the data matrix of six by four represents averaged ratings, the average measure ICC should be reported. Note that an internal consistency measure, α, estimate is identical to the ICC average = .9093.

```
             RELIABILITY   ANALYSIS   -   SCALE (ALPHA)

                     Analysis of Variance

Source of Variation    Sum of Sq.  DF   Mean Square    F       Prob.

Between People          56.2083     5     11.2417    31.8665   .0000
Within People          112.7500    18      6.2639
  Between Measures       97.4583     3     32.4861
  Residual               15.2917    15      1.0194
Total                  168.9583    23      7.3460
        Grand Mean        5.2917

              Intraclass Correlation Coefficient

Two-Way Random Effect Model (Consistency Definition):
People and Measure Effect Random
   Single Measure Intraclass Correlation = .7148*
    95.00% C.I.: Lower = .3425    Upper = .9459
     F = 11.0272  DF = (5,15.0)    Sig. = .0001 (Test Value = .0000 )
   Average Measure Intraclass Correlation = .9093
    95.00% C.I.: Lower = .6757    Upper = .9859
     F = 11.0272  DF = (5,15.0)    Sig. = .0001 (Test Value = .0000 )

*: Notice that the same estimator is used whether the interaction
effect is present or not.

Reliability Coefficients

N of Cases = 6.0
N of Items = 4
Alpha = .9093
```

A graphical illustration of how to use SPSS to calculate ICC is given in the file *COMPUTERILLUSTRATIONS 1* on the companion CD.

6.   Summary and Outlook

In this text, methods of rater agreement have been presented that operate at
the level of *manifest* variables, that is, at the level of observed variables.
Four groups of methods were discussed. First, using coefficients such as
Cohen's κ or its variants, one can condense information and concisely
describe the degree of agreement, using just one coefficient. In addition,
one can answer the question as to whether the agreement between two
raters goes beyond the agreement one would expect based on chance.
Chance models can be specified that reflect the assumptions made about the
process that determine agreement (cf. von Eye, & Sörensen, 1991; Zwick,
1988).

The second group of methods includes log-linear models. Using
these models, one can specify and test very detailed hypotheses concerning
agreement. A family of models was presented and discussed that
decomposes the joint frequency distribution of raters' judgements in four
components. The first component is the *base model*. This model typically
contains the intercept and the main effects of the variables that span the
cross-classification under study. The second component, represented by the
δ parameter, represents the *agreement cells*, that is, the cells in the main
diagonal. If the weights are equal, δ can be interpreted as an indicator of
strength of agreement. Differential weights can be used that reflect the
relative importance raters assign to individual categories.

The third component, represented by the β parameter, reflects *scale
characteristics of the rating categories*. If these categories are ordinal, a
linear-by-linear interaction term can be taken into account. This term

captures the variability carried by the ordinal nature of variables. Without this term, the models needed to explain the joint frequency distribution of ordinal variables can become unnecessarily complex.

The fourth component allows researchers to take *continuous covariates* into account. Covariates can come in many forms. Examples include average scores on independent variables that may have an effect on rating behavior, or probabilities for certain behaviors, and trends in cross-classifications, for example the trend of one of the raters to issue higher scores. The effects of covariates can be assessed by comparing models with covariates and models without covariates. Categorical covariates can be taken into account in the form of stratification variables.

The third group of methods for the analysis of rater agreement presented here is exploratory in nature. Using Configural Frequency Analysis (CFA), it was shown how cross-classifications of two or more raters' judgements can be explored, and those cells in which raters agree beyond chance identified as well as those cells in which raters disagree beyond chance. Covariates can be entertained, and the scale level of the rating categories can be taken into account. In addition, composite hypotheses can be explored.

The fourth group of methods comes with a change in perspective. Here, we no longer ask questions that can be answered by analyzing frequency tables. Instead, we ask whether the correlation matrices that can be calculated for variables used to describe behavior are specific for comparison objects. More specifically, if raters describe behavior using the same variables, these methods allows one to compare the group-specific correlation matrices.

There exists a number of alternative models and approaches to analyzing rater agreement. Three of these will be briefly reviewed here. The first approach involves *latent class modeling* (Agresti, 1992; Uebersax, 1993). In a fashion comparable to factor models, latent class models explain the covariation of categorical variables from unobserved (latent) variables. If the latent variables allow one to explain the covariation of categorical variables, these variables are statistically independent at each level of the latent class (cf. Bartholomew & Knott, 1999). Agresti (1992) illustrates latent class models for rater agreement using the three Raters A, B, and C. The cross-classification of these three raters' judgements has I x I x $I = I^3$ cells, where I denotes the number of rating categories used. Using a latent class model, researchers assume there exists an unobserved categorical variable, $X,^9$ that has L categories. The cases (judgements) in each of the L categories are homogeneous. Thus, the judgements provided by the Raters A, B, and C are statistically independent at each of the L levels of X, because X explains the covariation of the raters' judgements.

To describe the latent class model, let π_{ijkl} be the probability of a judgement by the three raters A, B, and C, in class l of the latent variable X, where i, j, and k index the rating categories used by the three raters, with $i, j, k, = 1, ..., I$. Suppose that N objects are rated. Then, the expected cell frequencies of the A x B x C x X cross-classification are estimated as $\hat{m}_{ijkl} = N\pi_{ijkl}$. The observed frequencies, $m_{ijk.}$, can be interpreted as the cell frequencies of the cross-classification of A, B, and C that was collapsed over the L categories of the latent variable, X. The log-linear model for the three raters and the latent variable, X, is

$$\log m = \lambda_0 + \lambda_i^A + \lambda_j^B + \lambda_k^C + \lambda_l^X + \lambda_{il}^{AX} + \lambda_{jl}^{BX} + \lambda_{kl}^{CX} .$$

Thus, this model proposes that the frequency distribution in the A x B x C x X cross-classification can be explained from the main effects of all four variables and the two-way interactions of the three observed variables with the latent variable. If individual observers' ratings are associated with X, the marginal associations between pairs of observers can be strong.

One option is to set $L = I$ for the number of latent classes, and to interpret the latent classes in a fashion parallel to the categories of the scale used by the raters. Then, the following probabilities are of interest:

(1) $p(A = i|X = i)$: the probability that Rater A indicates Category i given that the latent variable assumes the score i;

(2) $p(B = i|X = i)$: the probability that Rater B indicates Category i given that the latent variable assumes the score i; and

(3) $p(C = i|X = i)$: the probability that Rater C indicates Category i given that the latent variable assumes the score i.

One can also estimate probabilities of latent classes, conditioned on patterns of observed ratings. For example, one can ask what the probability is for latent Class i, given that Rater A indicated Category i, Rater B indicated Category j, and Rater C indicated Category k. Based on

---

[9] Note that in this section, X no longer denotes a design matrix but rather a latent variable.

these probabilities one can estimate the probability with which an object belongs to a particular latent class.

Latent class and latent trait models allow one to test hypotheses concerning rater effects. These effects are often rater characteristics such as rater cognition and the relationship between rater cognitive processing and rater proficiency. In addition, hypotheses can be tested concerning rater-specific accuracy and inaccuracy, rater-specific trends such as harshness or leniency (see Section 2.4.2), and centrality versus extremism (see Wolfe, 2004).

One problem with latent class models for rater agreement is that the number of estimated parameters is large. Often, models are not identified and one has to reduce the number of parameters to be estimated by setting some equal to zero or by setting some equal to each other. Placing such constraints is not arbitrary and results depend on these decisions. For binary rating variables, a minimum of three raters is necessary for a model to be identified.[10]

Extensions of the latent class model allow researchers to (1) model ordinal variables; (2) consider the latent variable continuous (latent trait models; see Bartholomew & Knott, 1999; Uebersax, 1993); (3) assume quasi-symmetry for the distribution among the observed judgements implied by a latent class model; and (4) consider Rasch models (cf. Lindsay, Clogg, & Grego, 1991).

The second alternative approach to be reviewed here briefly involves using models that assume that raters are fallible (Bakeman, Quera, McArthur, & Robinson, 1997). These models allow one to take into account the random component in raters' judgements.

The third group of methods comes from a different perspective than any of the models discussed in this text. DeCarlo (2004) proposes a latent class extension of signal detection theory that allows on to test a theory of psychological processes that underlie raters' behavior. This approach has the advantage of providing measures of the precision of raters and the accuracy of classifications. First applications in the area of essay grading have been presented (DeCarlo, 2004).

---

[10] Note that, in log-linear models of rater agreement, the number of parameters to be estimated can also exceed the number of available degrees of freedom (see Section 2.3.3.1).

References

Agresti, A. (1988). A model for agreement between ratings on an ordinal scale. *Biometrics, 44*, 539-548.

Agresti, A. (1992). Modeling patterns of agreement and disagreement. *Statistical Methods in Medical Research, 1*, 201-218.

Agresti, A. (1996). *An introduction to categorical data analysis.* New York: Wiley.

Agresti, A. (2002). *Categorical data analysis* (2nd ed.). New York: Wiley.

Agresti, A., Ghosh, A., & Bini, M. (1995). Raking kappa: Describing potential impact of marginal distributions on measures of agreement. *Biometrical Journal, 37*, 811-820.

Bakeman, R., Quera, V., McArthur, D., & Robinson, B. F. (1997). Detecting sequential patterns and determining their reliability with fallible observers. *Psychological Methods, 2*, 357-370.

Barnhart, H., & Williamson, J. M. (2002). Weighted least-squares approach for comparing correlated kappa. *Biometrics, 58*, 1012-1019.

Bartholomew, D. J., & Knott, M. (1999). *Latent variable models and factor analysis* (2nd ed.). London: Arnold.

Bishop, Y. M. M., Fienberg, S. E., & Holland, P. W. (1975). *Discrete multivariate analysis. Theory and practice.* Cambridge, MA: MIT Press.

Bortz, J., Licnert, G. A., & Boehnke, K. (1990). *Verteilungsfreie Methoden in der Biostatistik [distribution-free methods in biostatistics].* Berlin: Springer-Verlag.

Brennan, R. L., & Prediger, D. J. (1981). Coefficient kappa: Some uses, misuses, and alternatives. *Educational and Psychological Measurement, 41*, 687-699.

Cantor, A. B. (1996). Sample-size calculations for Cohen's kappa. *Psychological Methods, 1*, 150-153.

Christensen, R. (1997). *Log-linear models and logistic regression.* (2nd ed.). New York: Springer.

Cicchetti, D. V., & Allison, T. (1971). A new procedure for assessing reliability of scoring EEG sleep recordings. *American Journal of EEG Technology, 11*(3), 101-110.

Clogg, C. C., & Shihadeh, E. S. (1994). *Statistical models for ordinal variables.* Thousand Oaks, CA: Sage.

Cohen, J. (1960). A coefficient of agreement for nominal scales. *Educational and Psychological Measurement, 20*, 37-46.

Cohen, J. (1968). Weighted kappa: Nominal scale agreement with provision for scaled disagreement or partial credit. *Psychological Bulletin, 70,* 213-220.

Coleman, J. S. (1966). *Measuring concordance in attitudes.* Unpublished manuscript, Johns Hopkins University, Department of Social Relations.

Darlington, R. B., & Hayes, A. F. (2000). Combining independent p-values: Extensions of the Stouffer and binomial models. *Psychological Methods, 5,* 496-515.

DeCarlo, L. T. (2004). A model of rater behavior in essay grading based on signal detection theory. *Journal of Educational Measurement* (in press).

Donner, A., & Eliasziw, M. (1992). A goodness of fit approach to inference procedures for the kappa statistic: Confidence interval estimation, significance testing and sample size estimation. *Statistics in Medicine, 11,* 1511-1519.

DuMouchel, W. (1999). Bayesian data mining in large frequency tables, with an application to the FDA spontaneous reporting system. *The American Statistician, 53,* 177-190.

Everitt, B. S. (1998). *Dictionary of statistics.* Cambridge, UK: Cambridge University Press.

Evers, M., & Namboodiri, N. K. (1978). On the design matrix strategy in the analysis of categorical data. In K. F. Schuessler (Ed.), *Sociological methodology* (pp. 86-111). San Francisco, CA: Jossey-Bass.

Feinstein, A. R., & Cicchetti, D. V. (1990). High agreement but low kappa I: The problems of two paradoxes. *Journal of Clinical Epidemiology, 43,* 543-549.

Finkelstein, J. W., von Eye, A., & Preece, M. A. (1994). The relationship between aggressive behavior and puberty in normal adolescents: A longitudinal study. *Journal of Adolescent Health, 15,* 319-326.

Flack, V. F., Afifi, A. A., & Lachenbruch, P. A. (1988). Sample size determinations for the two rater kappa statistic. *Psychometrika, 53,* 321-325.

Fleiss, J. L. (1975). Measuring agreement between two judges in the presence or absence of a trait. *Biometrics, 31,* 651-659.

Fleiss, J. L. (1981). *Statistical methods for rates and proportions* (2nd ed.). New York: Wiley.

Fleiss, J. L., Cohen, J., & Everitt, B. S. (1969). Large sample standard errors of kappa and weighted kappa. *Psychological Bulletin, 72,* 323-327.

Froman, T., & Llabre, J. H. (1985). The equivalence of Kappa and Del. *Perceptual and Motor Skills, 60,* 651-659.

Furman, W., Simon, V. A., Shaffer, L., & Bouchey, H. A. (2002). Adolescents' working models and styles for relationships with parents, friends, and romantic partners. *Child Development, 73*(1), 241-255.

Glück, J., & von Eye, A. (2000). Including covariates in Configural Frequency Analysis. *Psychologische Beiträge, 42,* 405-417.

Goodman, L. A. (1979). Simple models for the analysis of association in cross-classifications having ordered categories. *Journal of the American Statistical Association, 74,* 537-552.

Goodman, L. A. (1984). *The analysis of cross-classified data having ordered categories.* Cambridge, MA: Harvard University Press.

Goodman, L. A., & Kruskal, W. H. (1954). Measures of association for cross-classifications. *Journal of the American Statistical Association, 49,* 732-764.

Graham, P. (1995). Modeling covariate effects in observer agreement studies: The case of nominal scale agreement. *Statistics in Medicine, 14,* 299-310.

Guggenmoos-Holzmann, I. (1995). Modeling covariate effects in observer agreement studies: The case of nominal scale agreement (letter to the editor). *Statistics in Medicine, 14,* 2285-2286.

Havránek, T., & Lienert, G.A. (1984). Local and regional versus global contingency testing. *Biometrical Journal, 26,* 483-494.

Hildebrand, D. K., Laing, J. D., & Rosenthal, H. (1977a). *Prediction analysis of cross-classifications.* New York: Wiley.

Hildebrand, D. K., Laing, J. D., & Rosenthal, H. (1977b). *Analysis of ordinal data.* Newbury Park: Sage.

Hommel, G. (1988). A stagewise rejective multiple test procedure based on a modified Bonferroni test. *Biometrika, 75,* 383-386.

Hommel, G., Lehmacher, W., & Perli, H. -G. (1985). Residuenanalyse des Unabhängigkeitsmodells zweier kategorialer Variablen [residual analysis of the independence model of two categorical variables]. In J. Jesdinsky & J. Trampisch (Eds.), *Prognose- und Entscheidungsfindung in der Medizin* (pp. 494-503) [*Making prognoses and decisions in medicine*]. Berlin: Springer.

Hsu, L. M., & Field, R. (2003). Interrater agreement measures: Comments on kappa$_n$, Cohen's kappa, Scott's π, and Aickin's α. *Understanding Statistics, 2,* 205-219.

Indurkhya, A., & von Eye, A. (2000). The power of tests in Configural

Frequency Analysis. *Psychologische Beiträge, 42*, 301-308.

Indurkhya, A., Zayas, L. H., & Buka, S. L. (2004). Sample size estimates for inter-rater agreement studies. *Methods of Psychological Research-online*. (in press)

Jackson, K. M., Sher, K. J., Gotham, H. J., & Wood, P. K. (2001). Transitioning into and out of large-effect drinking in young adulthood. *Journal of Abnormal Psychology, 110*(3), 378-391.

Jöreskog, K. G., & Sörbom, D. (1993). *LISREL 8 user's reference guide*. Chicago: Scientific Software International.

Kendall, M. G. (1962). *Rank correlation methods* (3rd ed.). London: Griffin.

Keselman, H. J., Cribbie, R., & Holland, B. (1999). The pairwise multiple comparison multiplicity problem: an alternative approach to familywise and comparisonwise Type I error control. *Psychological Methods, 4*, 58-69.

Kieser, M., & Victor, N. (1999). Configural frequency analysis (CFA) revisited-a new look at an old approach. *Biometrical Journal, 41*, 967-983.

Kirk, R. E. (1995). *Experimental design. Procedures for the behavioral sciences* (3rd ed.). Pacific Grove, CA: Brooks/Cole.

Kline, R. B. (1998). *Principles and practice of structural equation modeling*. New York: Guilford.

Landis, J. R., & Koch, G. G. (1977). The measurement of observer agreement for categorical data. *Biometrics, 33*, 159-174.

Lawal, H. B. (2001). Modeling symmetry models in square contingency tables with ordered categories. *Journal of Statistical Computing and Simulation, 71*, 59-83.

Lawal, H. B. (2003). *Categorical data analysis with SAS and SPSS applications*. Mahwah, NJ: Lawrence Erlbaum Associates.

Li, C. J., & Li, J. J. (2003). *The concordance correlation coefficient estimated through variance components*. IX Conference Española de Biometria.

Liebetrau, A. M. (1983). *Measures of association*. Beverly Hills, CA: Sage.

Lienert, G. A. (1978). *Verteilungsfreie Methoden in der Biostatistik*. (Vol. II) [*distribution-free methods in biostatistics*]. Meisenheim am Glan: Hain.

Lienert, G. A., & Krauth, J. (1975). Configural frequency analysis as a statistical tool for defining types. *Educational and Psychological Measurement, 35*, 231-238.

Light, R. J. (1969). *Analysis of variance for categorical data, with applications to agreement and association.* Unpublished dissertation, Harvard University, Department of Statistics.

Lindsay, B., Clogg, C. C., & Grego, J. (1991). Semiparametric estimation in the Rasch model and related exponential response models, including a simple latent class model for item analysis. *Journal of the American Statistical Association, 86*, 96-107.

McGraw, K. O., & Wong, S. P. (1996). Forming inferences about some intraclass correlation coefficients. *Psychological Methods, 1*, 30-46.

Meiser, T., von Eye, A., & Spiel, C. (1997). Log-linear symmetry and quasi-symmetry models for the analysis of change. *Biometrical Journal, 39*, 351-368.

Neter, J., Kutner, M. H., Nachtsheim, C. J., & Wasserman, W. (1996). *Applied linear statistical models* (4th ed.). Chicago: Irwin.

O'Connor, T. G., & Rutter, M. (1996). Risk mechanisms in development: Some conceptual and methodological considerations. *Developmental Psychology, 32*, 787-795.

Ohannessian, C. M., Lerner, R. M., Lerner, J. V., von Eye, A. (1995). Discrepancies in adolescents' and parents' perceptions of family functioning and adolescent emotional adjustment. *The Journal of Early Adolescence, 15*, 490-516.

Ohannessian, C. M., Lerner, R. M., Lerner, J. V., & von Eye, A. (2000). Adolescent-parent discrepancies in perceptions of family functioning and early adolescent self-competence. *International Journal of Behavioral Development, 24*, 362-372.

Pearson, K. (1901). Mathematical distributions to the theory of evolution. *Philosophical Transactions of the Royal Society of London (Series A) 197*, 385-497.

Perli, H. -G., Hommel, G., & Lehmacher, W. (1985). Sequentially rejective test procedures for detecting outlying cells in one- and two-sample multinomial experiments. *Biometrical Journal, 27*, 885-893.

Pugesek, B., Tomer, A., & von Eye, A. (2003), *Structural equation modeling: applications in ecological and evolutionary biology.* Cambridge, UK: Cambridge University Press.

Rae, G. (1988). The equivalence of multirater kappa statistics and intraclass correlation coefficients. *Educational and Psychological Measurement, 48*, 921-933.

Rudas, T. (1998). *Odds ratios in the analysis of contingency tables.* Thousand Oaks, CA: Sage.

SAS Institute Inc. (1999). *The SAS System for Windows* (version 8). Cary,

NC.

Schuster, C. (2001). Kappa as a parameter of a symmetry model for rater agreement. *Journal of Educational and Behavioral Statistics, 26,* 331-342.

Schuster, C., & von Eye, A. (2001). Models for ordinal agreement data. *Biometrical Journal, 43,* 795-808.

Shrout, P. E., & Fleiss, J. L. (1979). Intraclass correlations: Uses in assessing rater reliability. *Psychological Bulletin, 86,* 420-428.

Siegel, S. (1956). *Nonparametric statistics for the behavioral sciences.* New York: McGraw-Hill.

SPSS Inc. (2001). *SPSS for Windows* (version 11). Chicago, IL.

Stouffer, S. A., Suchman, E. A., DeVinney, L. C., Star, S. A., & Williams, R. M. Jr. (1949). *The American soldier: Adjustment during Army life* (Vol. 1). Princeton, NJ: Princeton University Press.

SYSTAT Software Inc. (2002). *SYSTAT for Windows* (version 10.2). Richmond, CA.

Tanner, M. A., & Young, M. A. (1985). Modeling agreement among raters. *Journal of the American Statistical Association, 80,* 175-180.

Uebersax, J. S. (1993). Statistical modeling of expert ratings on medical treatment appropriateness. *Journal of the American Statistical Association, 88,* 421-427.

Vermunt, J. K. (1997). Lem: *A general program for the analysis of categorical data.* Tilburg University.

von Eye, A. (1997). Prediction analysis program for 32 bit operation systems. *Methods for Psychological Research-online, 2,* 1-3.

von Eye, A. (2001). Configural Frequency Analysis (version 2000) program for 32 bit operating systems. *Methods of Psychological Research-Online, 6,* 129-139.

von Eye, A. (2002a). *Configural Frequency Analysis-methods, models, and applications.* Mahwah, NJ: Lawrence Erlbaum Associates.

von Eye, A. (2002b). The odds favor antitypes - A comparison of tests for the identification of configural types and antitypes. *Methods of Psychological Research-online, 7,* 1-29.

von Eye, A., & Mun, E. Y. (2004a). *Exploring rater agreement.* (in prep.).

von Eye, A. (2004b). *Base models for Configural Frequency Analysis.* (in prep.).

von Eye, A., & Brandtstädter, J. (1988a). Formulating and testing developmental hypotheses using statement calculus and non-parametric statistics. In P. B. Baltes, D. Featherman, & R. M. Lerner (Eds.), *Life-span development and behavior* (Vol. 8, pp. 61-

97). Hillsdale, NJ: Lawrence Erlbaum Associates.

von Eye, A., & Brandtstädter, J. (1988b). Application of prediction analysis to cross-classifications of ordinal data. *Biometrical Journal, 30,* 651-655.

von Eye, A., & Brandtstädter, J. (1998). The Wedge, the Fork, and the Chain - Modeling dependency concepts using manifest categorical variables. *Psychological Methods, 3,* 169-185.

von Eye, A., & Fuller, B. E. (2003). A comparison of the SEM software packages LISREL, EQS, and Amos. In B. Pugesek, A. Tomer, & A. von Eye (Eds.), *Structural equation modeling: Applications in ecological and evolutionary biology* (pp. 355-391). Cambridge, UK: Cambridge University Press.

von Eye, A., Jacobson, L. P., & Wills, S. D. (1990, May). *Proverbs: Imagery, interpretation, and memory.* Twelveth West Virginia University Conference on Life-Span Developmental Psychology.

von Eye, A., & Niedermeier, K. E. (1999). *Statistical analysis of longitudinal categorical data in the social and behavioral sciences.* Mahwah, NJ: Lawrence Erlbaum Associates.

von Eye, A., & Schuster, C. (1998a). On the specification of models for Configural Frequency Analysis - Sampling schemes in Prediction CFA. *Methods of Psychological Research-online, 3,* 55-73.

von Eye, A., & Schuster, C. (1998b). *Regression analysis for social sciences.* San Diego: Academic Press.

von Eye, A., & Schuster, C. (2000). Log-linear models for rater agreement. *Multiciência, 4,* 38-56.

von Eye, A., & Sörensen, S. (1991). Models of chance when measuring interrater agreement with kappa. *Biometrical Journal, 33,* 781-787.

Wickens, T. (1989). *Multiway contingency tables analysis for the social sciences.* Hillsdale, NJ: Lawrence Erlbaum Associates.

Willkinson, L. (2000). *SYSTAT for Windows* (version 10). Chicago: SPSS.

Wolfe, E. W. (2004). Identifying rater effects using latent trait models. *Psychology Science* (in press).

Wong, S. P., & McGraw, K. O. (1999). Confidence intervals and *F* tests for intraclass correlations based on three-way random effects models. *Educational and Psychological Measurement, 59,* 270-288.

Zwick, R. (1988). Another look at rater agreement. *Psychological Bulletin, 103,* 374-378.

Author Index

Subject Index

Printed and bound by CPI Group (UK) Ltd, Croydon, CR0 4YY

24/10/2024

01778600-0001